Ashtanga Yoga

Beginners Course Manual for Teachers

Dr Monica Gauci
Chiropractor

Published by Kaivalya Publications
PO Box 181
Crabbes Creek NSW 2483, Australia

© Monica Gauci 2010

This book is copyright. Apart from any fair dealing for the purposes of private study, research, criticism or review, as permitted under the Copyright Act, no part may be reproduced by any process without written permission from the author.

First published 2010

Illustrations by John Scott

Gauci, Monica.
Ashtanga Yoga Beginners Course Manual for Teachers
A step-by-step guide with a word-for-word detailed script on how to safely and effectively teach Ashtanga Yoga to beginners
1st ed.
ISBN: 978-0-9775126-9-0

This manual does not constitute medical advice. Contact a medical practitioner to determine whether you are fit to perform these yogic exercises. Yoga *asana* cannot be learned from media such as this manual, which is not able to give feedback, but must be learned from a qualified teacher. This manual can be used only for study and as a supplement to personal instruction. It is offered as additional education for teachers. It is aimed at the average student, who exists only in theory. In reality the teacher has to adapt the practice to the individual. Although yoga has manifold therapeutic benefits, the yoga described here is not specifically designed for the alleviation of diseases.

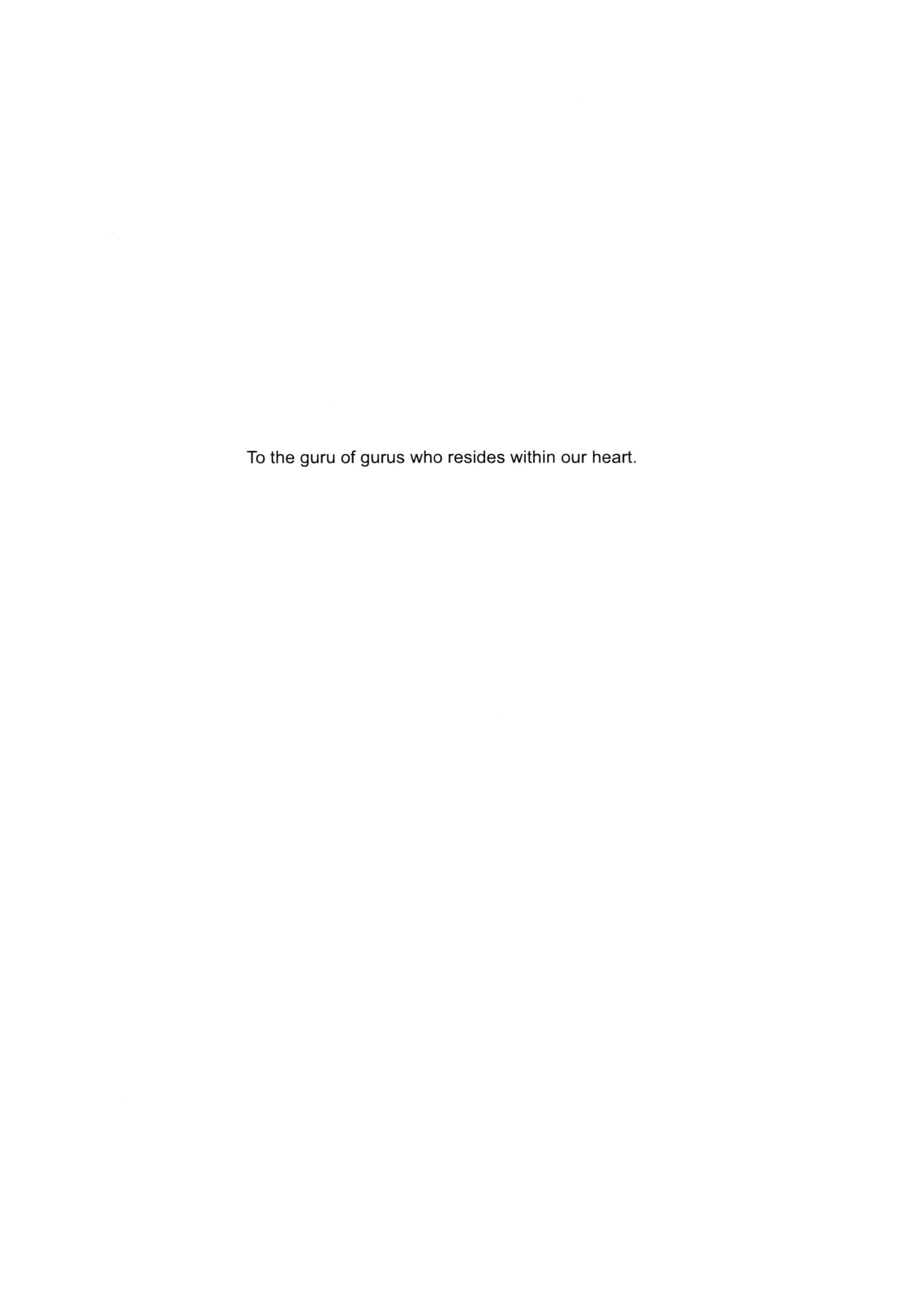

To the guru of gurus who resides within our heart.

TABLE OF CONTENTS

Acknowledgements	vi
Foreword by Gregor Maehle	vii

How To Use This Manual — 1

Week 1 • Learning to Breathe — 5

Welcome & Introduction	5
Pranayama & Diaphramatic Breathing	5
Ujjayi Pranayama	9
Samasthiti	10
Synchronising Breath with Movement	12
Surya Namaskara A	14
Padangushtasana	23
Breath Meditation	24
Shavasana	26

Week 2 • The Energy System — 31

Bandhas	32
Surya Namaskara B	34
Trikonasana	45
Yoga Mudrasana	47
Jnana Mudra	48
Uttpluthi	49

Week 3 • Drishti & Awareness — 53

Drishti	53
Talk-Through: Standing Postures	56
Parshvakonasana Modification	57
Prasarita Padottanasana A, B, C & D	59
Vinyasa Basic	62

Week 4 • The 8 Limbs — 67

8 Limbs of Yoga	67
Lowering Down in Sun Salutations	69
Parshvottanasana	71
Utthita Hasta Padangushtasana Preparation	75
Warrior Sequence	76
Vinyasa Stepping	80

Week 5 • Strength & Endurance — 85

Hopping in Sun Salutations		85
Hopping in Standing Postures		87
Dandasana		88
Pashimottanasana A & B		89
Purvottanasana		90
Vinyasa Stepping Back		93
Janu Shirshasana A		94
Janu Shirshasana B		96

Week 6 • The Flow of the Practice — 101

Talk-Through: Surya Namaskara A		102
Talk-Through: Surya Namaskara B		105
Talk-Through: Padangushtasana To UHP Preparation		109
Talk-Through: Warrior Sequence		114
Vinyasa Hopping To Sitting		116
Vinyasa Hopping Back From Sitting		119
Marichyasana A		122
Marichyasana C		124
Navasana		126

ACKNOWLEDGEMENTS

My thanks and gratitude to all my teachers who have taught me to learn and to develop the awareness to teach myself and refine my yoga practice.

A special thanks to my husband and devoted yogi Gregor Maehle for his outstanding contribution to my understanding of yoga philosophy. You are a constant inspiration and treasured companion on my yogic and life path.

Thank you to Carmela Lacey for her contribution, especially in the area of alternatives for students for some of the challenging aspects of the postures.

Acknowledgement and thanks to John Scott for his timeless illustrations of the Ashtanga Vinyasa Yoga postures.

And a big thank you to all our teachers and students at 8 Limbs in Perth, Australia and our teacher trainees worldwide for affording me the opportunity to teach and learn from you.

FOREWORD

The yoga conventionally called *Ashtanga Yoga* bears a great promise. The original Ashtanga or eight-limbed yoga is the yoga of the ancient Indian sage Patanjali and was already mentioned in scriptures such as the Mahabharata or the Shrimad Bhagavatam. In this mother of all yogas, posture (asana) is used as the foundation to support all other higher yogic techniques such as pranayama and meditation.

Unfortunately today Ashtanga Yoga is often misunderstood as a mere physical practice and limited to body-building and beautifying. Additionally its linear presentation lends itself to an attitude of conquering one posture after another and a mindset of acquisition and physical performance. But this practice offers so much more than mere posture-grabbing. To be true to its ancient roots it calls to be presented in an intelligent and compassionate way, guiding the student away from ambition and competition to enable him or her to eventually go beyond the body towards the spiritual practices. To achieve this it cannot be allowed to harm the body. Unfortunately much of today's discussions on yoga are related to the physical problems of yogis, which they have acquired through ambitious practice. Ambitious practice is often caused by teachers placing physical achievement into the focus of yoga students. With this fresh presentation of Ashtanga Vinyasa Yoga, outlined in this manual, we believe to have avoided these common pitfalls.

Hip Opening

The Ashtanga Vinyasa sequences as they are conventionally presented were designed for the ancient Indian people, who grew up sitting on the floor rather than on chairs. When sitting since a young age, when your joints are still pliable, in a cross-legged sitting position on the floor, the hip joints will naturally open as gravitation draws the knees downwards. When teaching students who grew up sitting on chairs, this needs to be taken into consideration. If failing to do so and students are forced into postures like lotus-posture, knee injuries may occur, typically injuries of the medial meniscus. When asked by the student for an explanation, a teacher not steeped in anatomy may escape to terminologies such as 'opening of the knees' to label something that is simply an injury. This constitutes himsa (violence) on the part of the teacher. It is not the knee joints that need to open, in fact the knee joints need to remain as taut as possible to keep its functional integrity. Instead, what needs to open is the hip joint.

A Three-layered Approach

Conventional Ashtanga practice needs to be modified for modern students who often start out with very stiff hip joints. Otherwise the knee joints have to make up for the lack of flexibility that the hip joints have not yet acquired. Any postures that require more advanced hip opening can provoke knee injury, such as Janushirshasana C, Marichyasana D, Garbhapindasana, etc. These postures need to be initially removed from the syllabus and be presented only once the students' hip joints have acquired an increased range of motion to allow for such postures.

For safety purposes we present the Ashtanga practice in three layers:

1. Beginners Course Level 1 in which only those postures that are safe for all students are introduced. This excludes all posture that require increased hip rotation.

2. Beginners Course Level 2 adds postures that require moderate hip flexibility and can be practiced once the postures of Level 1 are learned. In this level Baddha Konasana is introduced. It helps the student to develop the ability to safely practice postures that come before it in the conventional Primary series.

3. Mysore-style class: Here the more difficult postures are added according to individual capabilities. These postures may come in the conventional series prior to some Level 1 and 2 postures but if presented in the order suggested here any potential harm is avoided and only the benefits are derived. There is no value in being 'traditional' if this harms your students and to avoid harming students (ahimsa) is the most important precept for the yoga teacher.

Importance of the Beginners Course Format

To be able to provide a student right from the beginning with lots of information one needs to initially depart from the so-called Mysore-style format. While the Mysore-style format is great for more experienced students, if applied right from the outset of teaching, it leads to a sloppy practice for most novice students. During Mysore-style classes the teacher cannot cater for the novices' need for detailed information regarding the practice in general and the individual postures in particular. The teacher in a Mysore-style class does not have the time available to talk to each novice for an hour and yet this amount of information is required to unleash the full potential of this practice. For this reason we have created a beginners course curriculum for all beginning students before they advance to Mysore-style classes. We found such a curriculum can be taught over a minimum of 12 classes delivered over two courses (Beginners Course Level 1 and 2) but it can also be spread over as many as 20 classes (Beginners Intensive Level 1 and 2) in which case even more attention to detail can be afforded. In this manual Monica Gauci presents the curriculum of our Level 1 Beginners Course, which has proven itself as the foundation of our teaching success. Implementing this curriculum in your yoga studio will lead to high-quality practice and minimize potential harm implied in the conventional presentation of Ashtanga Yoga.

Importance to Include Western Anatomy in Describing Postures

There are four ways of achieving proper alignment in yoga postures:

1. In the Vedic and Puranic method, which was practised by the ancient Indians, each asana has an underlying divine form. By meditating on the underlying divine form the yogi is able to experience the alignment of a particular posture. This is the most time intense method for modern westerners as it requires to not only understand Sanskrit phonetics and etymology but also to read the required scriptures. For example, when wanting to experience the alignment of Hanumanasana, one needs to study the Yuddhakanda of the Ramayana. Here Lord Hanuman spans in one giant leap the entire distance from the Himalayas to Sri Lanka to save the Lakshmana, the brother of Lord Rama. For someone who has not grown up in Hindu culture steeped in the many images of this incident, this method of experiencing alignment is not feasible.

2. The tantric method, used by siddhas like Gorakhnath is a reciprocal relationship between the alignment of subtle body and that of the gross body. When one focuses on entry of prana into sushumna and the alignment of its upper opening "Brahmarandhra" with the chakras on the soft palate, any faulty alignment of the gross body is immediately noticed. This is an advanced method and not accessible to novices.

3. Using the rehabilitation method, if you have an injury such as micro tears in the cartilage of the meniscus and are a sensible practitioner you can experiment with various versions of alignment. If your alignment was slightly faulty your body will give you feedback within the next eight hours. You can then slightly alter your alignment and compare the feedback after the next practice session. Through trial and error you will slowly arrive at the correct alignment. This method can yield highly precise results especially if the practitioner is sensible but it can only be used after the problem has occurred.

4. Through the Western anatomical method, the yoga teacher can research and understand range of joint movement and limitations of the human body in yoga postures. To do this you need an understanding of major muscles, ligaments, fascia, tendons, bones and joints. With these tools postures can be described in such a way that they become safe and the benefits are maximized. This is the easiest, safest and most straightforward method for modern yogis with the least amount of time involved. That there are still yoga teachers who refuse to use this tool just because it was not utilized by ancient yogis, is baffling.

Lots of Information

There is an old adage that says, 'People will make the best decision based on the information at hand.' If you want to improve the quality of decisions, you need to supply quantity and quality of information. In our beginners courses we endeavour to arm students with as much quality information on the fundamentals of yoga and the individual postures as possible. This enables students to make quality decisions in postures and progress faster with little or no setbacks. We found that this is best done from as early on as possible. Students who have not received sophisticated instruction on breath, bandhas and alignment right from the beginning, find it difficult later on to switch to a more refined form of practice. This is similar to a music or dance student. Once the student has settled into sloppy technique it is more difficult to change. However, it is easy to instill love of detail of alignment, breath and bandhas right from the beginning.

I believe that this manual compiled by my wife, Monica Gauci, will greatly aid your teaching and be of great benefit to your students.

Gregor Maehle

Internationally renown author of :

Ashtanga Yoga - Practice & Philosophy
Ashtanga Yoga -The Intermediate Series
Pranayama - The Breath of Yoga
Yoga Meditation - Through Mantra, Chakras and Kundalini to Spiritual Freedom

HOW TO USE THIS MANUAL

This manual came into creation as a resource and aid to help Yoga teachers-to-be to find the words to describe some of the techniques and asanas when teaching yoga. It is a modification of the Primary Series of Ashtanga Vinyasa Yoga, which deletes or modifies any postures which are not accessible to the average beginner student.

There are many approaches to teaching Ashtanga Vinyasa Yoga to beginners. I devised this approach over many years and over the last 17 years it has been successfully applied to thousands of yoga students as the basic 8 Limbs Beginners program in Perth, Australia and its lineage of teachers.

The program is set out over a six-week course, however, the same information also can easily be distributed over eight or more classes. Each class has been given a theme and an overview. The overview includes what is taught new in that class as well as what will need revising, i.e. what was taught new in the last class. It also includes a section of 'Notes', which draw the teacher trainee's attention to any important pointers for the topics covered in that class. Notes are also included for each posture and sometimes within the text of particular postures.

The teaching methods given include various alternatives and a multitude of instructions for each technique and asanas described. Obviously the possibilities are inexhaustible. These instructions are anatomically sound, thorough and balanced. Each topic and set of instructions is broken down into an 'Overview', an 'Introduction', a 'Demonstration', performing the posture with the student 'Do With' and watching the students do the posture 'Watch Them'. This 5-step format has proven to be a very effective teaching method of any yogic asana or technique. Overview, as the name suggests gives a summary of how the topic is presented with its own section of notes. For the demonstrations, directional suggestions are given for the best vantage position for the students observing. Minimal instruction is advised to maximise on visual learning. More extensive instructions are given when the posture is performed with students and a lavish array of descriptions are included in the section where the teacher is observing the students. Additional 'Workshop' sections are included as an analytical dissection of more complex or challenging postures or aspects of a posture. These instructions break down the individual components of a movement and put it 'under the microscope' to ensure that it is performed safely and effectively.

To further ensure safety and to build student confidence some postures have been entirely left out of the traditional Primary Series or have been modified. For example, the half-lotus postures have been removed and a preparation or variation of the full posture is given for Parshvakonasana and Utthita Hasta Padangustasana. Additionally, some drishtis have been modified. If the student chooses to progress with their Ashtanga Vinyasa Yoga practice, these modifications and deletions would be substituted in a Level 2 course.

Any teaching methodology stands or falls with the result it achieves. This present method has been distilled from many years of observing students practice and the influence certain ways of demonstrating and delivering instructions achieves. You will find that this method will achieve a high level of proficiency and quality in your student's performance, while adhering to the highest safety standards. With this comes the highest level of benefit for the student.

"A teacher affects eternity: he can never tell where his influence stops."

Henry Brooks Adams

Week 1

WEEK 1 • Learning to Breathe

Class Overview	<ul><li>Welcome and Introduction</li><li>Teach the breathing exercise</li><li>Teach *Ujjayi* sound</li><li>Teach *Samasthiti*</li><li>Teach synchronising breath with movement</li><li>Teach *Surya Namaskara A*</li><li>Teach *Padangustasana* and *Pada Hastasana*</li><li>Teach seated breath meditation<ul><li>Open cross-legged position</li></ul></li><li>Teach *Shavasana*</li></ul>**NOTE:**<ul><li>Whenever students are sitting for longer than a minute have them all seated on a blanket (eg. introduction and seated meditation)</li></ul>

Welcome & Introduction

	<ul><li>**Welcome and thank you for coming**</li><li>**Housekeeping**<ul><li>Shoe rack, toilets, change room, drinking water and mobiles switched off</li></ul></li><li>**Introduction to school/you and what makes you special**</li><li>**Commitment – yours and theirs**</li><li>**Punctuality**<ul><li>Importance of warm-up and introductory information</li></ul></li></ul>

Pranayama & Diaphragmatic Breathing

Overview	<ul><li>**Introduction of the breath, including:**<ul><li>The yogic importance of the breath</li><li>What *pranayama* is (either here or when *ujjayi* sound is introduced)</li><li>The physical importance of using the diaphragm<ul><li>Some options are given in the 'Introduction' section</li></ul></li></ul></li><li>**Demonstrate areas of the chest**</li><li>**Teach the breathing exercise**<ol><li>Students lie on their back</li><li>Observe their 'normal' breathing</li><li>Breath exercise with hands on each area of the chest in turn</li><li>Finish with a smooth flow between the areas</li><li>Sit students up to summarise the effect of the exercise</li></ol></li></ul>

	NOTE: • Walk around the students, using gentle touch as a correction as you continue to instruct the whole group • Conduct each breath for them – inhalation and exhalation • It is important to remind students to 'keep breathing' as you change areas if you want them to stay with you on every breath call • First breath is short, build up the length of each breath as each area is added on • Make your instruction match the length of each breath • Minimum of 5 breaths into each area • Remember to instruct students to breath in and out through their nose • Get students to keep their eyes open to keep them focused

Introduction	**The importance of the breath in yoga**
	• Yogis were the first to recognise the intimate relationship/connection between the breath and the mind
	• One of the most important discoveries that yogis made is that the breath effects the mind and vice versa
	   o Eg, when anxious breath becomes quick and shallow, when relaxed the breath is slow and deep
	   o The longest living animals are those that breathe the slowest!
	• Regulating your breath can calm/still your mind
	• The purpose of yoga ultimately is to still the mind
	
	The extension and/or control of the breath in yoga is called 'pranayama'
	• 'Prana' means life force - the breath carries our life force
	• 'Ayama' means extension
	
	The diaphragm muscle is the primary muscle of respiration
	• It is a flat muscle that attaches sits like a dome (use hands to show shape) at the bottom of our ribcage and separates the chest from the abdominal organs
	• When you breathe in/inhale the diaphragm descends, pushes the belly out and widens the ribcage circumferentially/horizontally
	• Various stresses cause people to not use their diaphragm muscle fully when breathing. Dysfunctional breathing can become habitual
	• Using the diaphragm muscle [options]
	   o Keeps the chest flexible
	   o Takes tension off the neck
	   o Strengthens the pelvic floor
	   o Strengthens the abdominal wall and low back
	   o Massages the abdominal organs and
	   o Has many other health benefits
	
	• We're going to do an exercise to develop our awareness of our breath and learn how to extend/expand our breath by using our diaphragm muscle fully
	• During the exercise I will ask you to place your hands on different areas of your chest

Demonstration	<ul><li>These are the areas of the chest:<ul><li>We'll call the 'front' of your chest this soft area low down on your rib cage between your last ribs</li><li>The 'sides' of your chest is where you can feel your ribs</li><li>The 'back' of your chest - you'll need to slip your hands under your back when we're lying down and</li><li>The 'top' of your chest is just below your collar bones</li></ul></li></ul>
Breathing Exercise	<ul><li>**Lie on Back**<ul><li>Lie down on your back and keep your eyes open</li><li>If it's more comfortable for you, you can bend your knees – take your feet apart and then let your knees fall in on each other until they are touching</li></ul></li><li>**Normal Breathing**<ul><li>Without changing how you are breathing, notice what happens when you inhale. Do your ribs move or spread or your belly rise up towards the ceiling? As you exhale the chest and abdomen should deflate.</li></ul></li><li>**Breathing Through the Nose**<ul><li>In yoga breathing is done in and out is through the nose – your mouth is for many other things but not for breathing!</li></ul></li><li>**Hands on Chest Areas**</li><li>**Front**<ul><li>Place one hand on the front of your chest<ul><li>Inhale into the front of your chest</li><li>Exhale out through the nose</li><li>Inhale so your hand rises</li><li>Exhale, feel the chest fall</li><li>Inhale into the area under your hand</li><li>Exhale through your nose</li><li>Inhale into the front of the chest</li><li>Exhale</li><li>Once more into your hands</li><li>And out through your nose</li></ul></li></ul></li><li>**Sides**<ul><li>Keep breathing and now move your hands to the side of your chest over your ribs OR</li><li>Keep breathing and now place both hands on the front of your chest so your fingertips interlace on the front of your chest and the heels of your hands rest on your ribs at the sides of your chest<ul><li>Inhale into the front and now into the sides of your chest where your hands are OR</li><li>Inhale into the front of the chest and now the sides so your fingertips slide past each other</li><li>Exhale to the same length as your inhalation</li><li>Inhale to the front of the chest, expand your breath to the sides</li><li>Exhale, controlling the breath as your breathe out</li><li>Inhale the front of the chest rises, the ribs expand</li><li>Exhale smoothly through your nose</li><li>Inhale into the front and now feel the ribs expand to the side</li><li>Exhale to the same length as your inhalation</li></ul></li></ul></li></ul>

- **Back**
    - Keep breathing. You can either leave your hands where they are or if it's comfortable, slip them under your chest so that the backs of your fingers touch the back of your chest
        - Inhale into the front, the sides and now breathe into the back of your chest
        - Exhale controlling the breath on the way out so that it remains smooth and long
        - Inhale feel the front of your chest rise, the sides expand and the back of your chest press into the mat/your hands
        - Exhale to the same length of time as your inhalation
        - Inhale into the front of your chest, the sides and now the back of your chest
        - Exhale through your nose, keep the breath smooth and long
- **Top**
    - Keep breathing and place your hands onto the top of your chest, just beneath your collar bones
        - Inhale into the front, the sides, the back and now the area beneath your hands at the top of your chest
        - Exhale smoothly and slowly matching the length of your exhalation to your inhalation
        - Inhale breathe into the front, the sides, the back and feel the top of your chest expand. Do not lift your chest to your chin
        - Exhale controlling the breath to be long and smooth
        - Inhale, the front of the chest rises, the ribs expand, the back presses into the mat and the top lobes of the lungs fill with breath
        - Exhale through your nose to the same length as your inhalation
- **Finish with a smooth flow between the four areas**
    - Place your hands on the mat beside you and continue breathing fully, deeply and smoothly
        - Inhale through your nose and notice how the breath naturally moves the front, the side and back and then the top of the chest
        - Exhale through your nose and notice how as the breath leaves the reverse action takes place
        - Inhale smoothly, fully and deeply
        - Exhale the same length as your inhalation
        - Inhale check that the top of the chest expands but does not rise up to your chin
        - Exhale
- **Summarise**
    - Roll over onto your side and push yourself up to come up to sitting
    - Did you notice that simply by using the diaphragm muscle fully you could lengthen and slow down your breath?
    - Breathing into all areas of the chest means we are breathing fully
    - Are there any questions on diaphragmatic breathing or *pranayama*?

Ujjayi Pranayama

Overview	- **Introduce *Ujjayi pranayama*** - **Teach how to make the sound** - **Demonstrate the sound** - **Do it with them and listen to them do it** **NOTE:** - This may be taught sitting or standing - Standing may make them less inhibited and makes it easier for you to listen to their breath as you walk around - Give as many instructions as possible while the students are doing the exercise versus in the introduction – see under 'Do With/ Watch Them'

Introduction	- In Ashtanga Yoga we use a particular breath system or style of *pranayama* where the breath is both full and directed.
	- This is called *Ujjayi pranayama* which means victorious stretching of the breath.
	- We've leant how to make the breath full by using the whole of our chest and we direct the breath by narrowing its passage
	  - For example, if you have 5 or 6 lanes of traffic it is more difficult to direct the flow compared to only one lane
	- We narrow the passage of the breath by constricting the muscles in our throat
	- This narrows the opening between our vocal cords (the glottis) and creates an aspirate/hissing/distinctive sound
	- The sound of the breath should be pleasant
	  - Some liken it to 'the wind in the trees', 'waves on a shore', or 'Darth Vader' whose breath is way too fast!

Demonstration	- The easiest way to get the *ujjayi* sound is to imitate it
	  - I'll walk around and make the sound for you
	- [Walk around your students making a loud, audible *ujjayi* sound]
	  - Could everyone hear that?
	
	Alternative
	- The action in your throat is the same as when you whisper
	- Imagine you are about to whisper something, then close your mouth and breath instead
	  - 'Hello my name is….., [close your mouth and make the *ujjayi* sound]

Do With / Watch Them	- Now it's your turn - Imitate the sound I am making - OR - Whisper 'Hello my name is….', then close your mouth, keep the same constriction in your throat and breath - Raise your hand if you're having problems and I'll come and help you

- [Walk around the students to listen and/or assist]
- The sound comes from your chest and not from your nose
- The sound of the inhalation and exhalation are the same
- At this stage, I want the sound of your breath to be so loud that I can hear you
  - With so many of you in the room it should sound like a storm in here!
  - From the sound of your breath I can judge the quality of your breathing
    - If the sound becomes harsh I know you are trying too hard or straining
    - If I don't hear you breathing I know you aren't focusing on your breathing/doing the *ujjayi pranayama*/you're about to collapse/die!
- Breathe in and out through your nose
- Breath into all four areas of your chest – the front, the sides, the back and the top of your chest
- Keep the breath full, feel your ribcage expand and deflate with your breath
- Listening to the breath helps to still and focus the mind, which is the original purpose of practicing yoga

---

Samasthiti	*drishti*: straight ahead or on the floor

Overview	• **Introduce *Samasthiti***
	 • **Do *Samasthiti* with them for the first few instructions only**
	 • **Watch and walk around them**
	
	 NOTE:
	 • Make their first *Samasthiti* very extensive
	    ○ Below are a variety of instructions that can be used
	       ■ Choose some or use your own words
	    ○ As the course progresses, *Samasthiti* can be less extensive
	 • Vary your script each time
	    ○ Both during each class and from class to class, to cover a wide variety of instructions
	 • Have a pattern or theme to make each total description balanced, eg:
	    ○ Work from the feet upwards
	    ○ Concentrate of one aspect, eg: weight distribution
	    ○ Juxtapose instructions, eg: as you ground down through your feet, grow up out of your insteps
	       ■ Choose from the instructions below to fit your theme
	 • Use gentle touch for individual corrections
	    ○ Whilst you continue to instruct the whole group
	 • Include the breathing and bandhas as they are introduced in each class

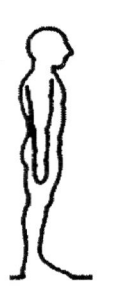

Introduction	- So lets come to standing and do our first yoga posture or asana
- This first posture we will be learning is the most important of the postures we will learn because
- It is correct posture and we will carry it into every other posture that we do
- All the actions you learn in this posture you will use in every other posture
- It is like a blueprint of how your posture should be
- It's called *Samasthiti* which means equal-standing or equal stance posture
Demonstrate face-on & side-on **Do With / Watch Them**	- To achieve 'equal-standing' we need to make sure that our weight is equally distributed in our feet
- Look down to your feet and stand with them together or as close as you can bring them together
- Imagine a line drawn from your second toe (the one alongside your big toe) through to the centre of your heel
- This is the 'straight line' of your foot – now check that your feet are straight
- Let your heels be slightly apart
- Become aware of the four corners of your feet: the base of your big toes, the base of your little toes and the inside and outside of each heel
- Distribute your weight equally between your feet and then the 4 corners of each foot
- As you ground the 4 corners of your feet, lift your insteps and feel your feet become strong and active/alive
- Let your feet become like suction pads, with the 4 outside corners gripping the mat and the insteps sucking up
- This lift from the insteps continues up the legs, lifting the knee caps as you contract your thighs or quads/quadriceps muscles
- Again this lift continues into the pelvis, along the entire length of your spine and neck, and up through the crown of your head
- Maintain this lift in the torso and feel as if your sit bones are heavy, anchoring the pelvis/like they have lead weights attached to them
- The lower abdomen is firm
- Contract your buttocks lightly, do not clench your buttocks until they harden
- Adjust your positioning so that your pelvis sits above your ankles, your shoulders above your hips and your ears back in line with your shoulders
- This will bring the weight of the body to fall just in front of the heels
- When your weight is evenly distributed your posture becomes light as there is the least resistance against gravity
- Let this lightness of posture be your guide
- The centre of your chest area we will call the 'heart' area, so lift your heart and let your chest spread in all four directions as you breathe
- Listen to the sound of your breath
- At the same time, loop your shoulders back and actively draw your shoulder blades down your back
- Be careful to not restrict the back of your chest when your breathe

	- Create space between your shoulder blades
	- Broaden the back of your chest
	- Keep the back of the heart open
	- Soften the lowest ribs back in /towards your torso
	  - Do not splay open the lower edge of the ribcage
	- Activate your arms all the way down to your fingers
	- Keep the hands soft
	- Drop your chin slightly so the front of the throat is soft
	- Lengthen the back of your neck
	- Grow the crown of your head upwards to the ceiling
	- Relax your face
	- Smooth your brow
	- Soften your gaze
	- Gaze straight ahead or at a spot on the floor out in front of you
	- Creating the *ujjayi* sound, check that your are breathing into the front, the sides, the back and the top of your chest
	- Keep directing the breath and breathing fully
	  - This is *Samasthiti*/the equal-standing posture
	  - We enter each standing posture via *Samasthiti* and return to it between each standing posture to resume our correct posture

Synchronising Breath with Movement

Overview	- **Introduce the concept of synchronising the breath with movement**
	- **Demonstrate**
	- **Do with them 3-5 times**
	  - The most basic instructions given here
	- **Watch them and give extra instructions 3-5 times**
	  - Each time add in another instruction
	  - Attempt to add in a different instruction with each repetition
	- **NOTE:**
	  - You may do some or all of the workshop themes here or otherwise they need be done in *Surya Namaskara A*

Introduction	- Over the course of the next few weeks we will be learning a sequence of warm up postures.
	- In Ashtanga Yoga every movement is synchronised with your breath.
	  - Every upward movement is done on an inhalation, every downward movement on an exhalation
	  - In fact, the breath initiates each movement
	- Watch me as I demonstrate

Demonstrate face-on	- For example, I breath in and raise my arms above my head
- As I exhale I lower my arms back down to my sides
- The movement should imitate your breath: smooth, slow, conscious, controlled
- Map your breath over the whole of the movement
- As I complete my inhalation my hands come together above my head
- As I complete my exhalation my hands come back to my sides
- Let's try that together
Do With/ Watch Them	- Inhale, turn your palms up, raise your arms above your head
- Exhale, palms down and lower your arms to your side
- Inhale, palms up, raise your arms, palms together above the head
- Exhale, palms down, lower your arms back down to your side
- Inhale, palms up, arms up, spread your breath over the whole movement
- Exhale, palms down, arms down, finish the exhale as your arms return to your side
- Inhale, stretching your breath long as you raise your arms, keep it smooth
- Exhale, control the breath out, spread it over the whole movement
- Inhale, keep your shoulders low and raise your arms, gaze up
- Inhale, shoulders heavy, light arms, palms together, look to your thumbs
- Inhale, arm straight and strong, shoulders down, gaze to the thumbs
- Inhale, turn the palms up, shoulders down, reach your arms up above your head, look up
- Inhale, lifting your chin at the same rate as your arms and gaze up
- Inhale, shoulders down, straight arms up, work the arms back towards your ears
- Inhale, shoulders down, straight arms up, lift your chin to gaze to your thumbs
Workshop	**Shoulders**
- Let me get a bit more specific with how to work our shoulders
- When you raise your arms up, be careful to not lift your shoulders
    - **[Demonstrate hunching shoulders, back-on]**
- You will need to actively draw the shoulders down away from your ears as you raise your arms OR
- You will need to actively draw your shoulder blades down your back as you raise your arms up

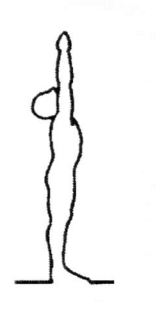

Arms
- **[Demonstrate, side-on]**
- Inhale, palms up, keep your arms straight as you raise them up
    - To keep your arms straight may mean that your hands end forward of your head
    - Once in this position work towards bringing your arms back towards your ears |

- Exhale, when you lower your arms keep them strong as if resisting against something on the way down
    - Try that

Neck
- **[Demonstrate, side-on]**
- At the same rate as you lift your arms, lift your chin so you end gazing up to your thumbs
- Be careful not to just throw/hang your head back but actively lift the chin up
    - Your neck is designed to extend back. We were meant to be able to look at the stars
        - Let's try that together

Flaring the Ribs
- When you raise your arms above your head check that you are not flaring open the bottom of your rib cage and arching backwards
- Watch me
    - **[Demonstrate wrong version, side-on]**
    - That's how you don't want to do it
- The position of your trunk should not change. Instead only the arms and the gaze are raised
    - **[Demonstrate, side-on]**
- As you raise your arms, anchor your lowest ribs/ribcage by using your abdominal muscles

Surya Namaskara A

Overview	

	- **Introduce Surya Namaskara**
	- **Break-down each move/vinyasa into**
	    - Demonstrate, do with them, watch them and workshop
	- **Teach Ekam to Chatvari (Rod)**
	    - Each time adding on from Samasthiti
	- **Teach Chatvari to Shat (Downward Dog)**
	    - Each time adding on from Chatvari (Rod)
	- **Combine Ekam to Shat (Downward Dog)**
	- **Teach from Shat to Samasthiti**
	- **Teach the complete Surya Namaskara A**
	    - Demonstrate, do one with them and watch them do two more
	
	NOTE:
	- You may also demonstrate a complete *Surya Namaskara* after the introduction
	- Beginners step back into the Rod
	- Beginners do the Rod with straight arms, i.e. without lowering down
	- Hold the first Rod and Upward Dog for a few breaths each
	- Take students into the child posture after Upward Dog
	- For safety reasons, some workshopping will need to be done before you do the posture with them

Introduction	- So this movement we've just done is actually part of the first sequence we will learn which a sun salutation
	  - In Sanskrit – the ancient language of India – the sun is called *Surya* and *Namaskara* or *Namaste* is a greeting
	  - *Surya Namaskara* is Sanskrit for sun salutation and it is a sequence of postures traditionally done to greet the rising sun
	  - Sun salutations strengthen the body and make it supple. They are also said to bring sunlight to the spirit
	- We'll learn each part separately and then put the whole thing together

Demonstration *Dve* side-on	- The first movement we already know
	  - Standing at the top end of your mat in *Samasthiti*
	  - Inhale, arms up, gaze to the thumbs, then
	
	Dve
	  - Exhale fold forward at the hips
	  - Knees bend
	  - Hands toward the floor
	  - Inhale, head comes up first, gaze up
	  - Exhale, *Samasthiti*

Workshop *Dve*
 	
Demonstration side-on
	- To protect your low back it is important to keep your low back from rounding. You can monitor this by keeping your lower abdomen in contact with your thighs. This will mean you will have to bend your knees as you fold forward
	  - Whenever we take the natural curve out of our low back it places stress on the discs between our vertebrae
	  - So let's try bending forward first with our hands on our hips so you can feel them tilt forward
	- When you do no longer feel your hips moving forward, bend your knees until your abdomen is on your thighs
	  - Let's do that together
	  - Inhale, lift up out of your feet, strong legs
	  - Exhale, fold forward
	    - Feel your hips tilt, when they stop bend your knees, low belly in contact with your thighs
	  - Take a few of breaths here/Keep breathing
	    - With your low belly close to your thighs, work towards straightening the legs until you feel a gentle stretch (on the hamstring muscles) in the back of your legs
	    - Spread your sit bones wide/Work the sit bones to the ceiling
	    - Relax and lengthen your spine and neck
	    - Shoulders lift away from your ears
	    - Drop your head
	  - Inhale, lift your head first, come all the way up to standing, arms above your head, look to your thumbs
	  - Exhale, arms down to *Samasthiti*

Dve
 	
Do With / Watch Them
	Add on from *Samasthiti*
	
	- Now let's add that on to our first move
	  - Standing at the top end of your mat in *Samasthiti*
	  - Inhale, arms up, shoulders down, look to the thumbs
	  - Exhale fold forward at the hips
	    - Bend your knees, fingers toward the floor
	  - Take a couple of breaths here
	    - Spread your sit bones wide
	    - Lengthen your spine and neck
	    - Drop your head
	  - Inhale, lift your head first, come all the way to upright, arms above your head, look to your thumbs
	  - Exhale, arms down to *Samasthiti*

Introduction & Demonstration side-on
 	
Trini
	- Let's add on the third move
	- I'll demonstrate it first
	  - From *Samasthiti*
	  - Inhale, arms up, look to the thumbs
	  - Exhale fold forward
	  - Inhale lift the chest, broad shoulders
	  - Exhale, fold forward again
	  - Inhale, come up, arms up
	  - Exhale back to *Samasthiti*

Trini **Do With / Watch Them**	**Add on from *Samasthiti*** - Standing at the top end of your mat in *Samasthiti* - Inhale, raise the arms up, shoulders heavy, look to the thumbs - Exhale bend your knees, fold forward, drop your head - Inhale lift your chest, shoulders down away from the ears - Exhale, fold down again, spread your sit bones wide/sit bones to the ceiling - Inhale, lift your head first, come all the way to up, arms above your head, look to your thumbs - Exhale, arms down to *Samasthiti*

Introduction & Demonstration side-on
 	
Chatvari (Rod)
	Step back into Rod; Rod with straight arms
	
	- Watch as I demonstrate the next posture we're going to add on
	- It's called the Rod and you'll soon see why
	  - From *Samasthiti*
	  - Inhale, arms up, look to the thumbs
	  - Exhale belly on thighs, fold forward
	  - Inhale lift the chest, shoulders down
	  - Exhale, step back into a long, strong, straight Rod
	  - Then come to your knees

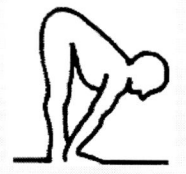

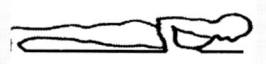

	Stepping Back Long [re-demonstrate from *Trini*]
	• When you step back into the Rod
	    o Keep your shoulders above your wrists
	    o Then step your right leg back as far as you can
	        ▪ Check that your buttocks are low, below the level of your shoulders
	    o Now step the left foot back to meet the right
	    o Position your feet hip-width apart

Do With / Watch Them	• Standing at the top of your mat in *Samasthiti* • Inhale, arms up, shoulders down, lift your chin to look to the thumbs • Exhale bend your knees, fold forward, drop your head • Inhale lift your heart, shoulders above your wrists • Exhale, step the right foot as far back as you can • Step the left back to meet it so you arrive in a long, strong Rod

Workshop *Chatvari*	**Straight Rod**
	• It's important to form a long, strong, straight Rod
	    o It's not the banana posture, or a camel
	        ▪ **[Demonstrate each, side-on]**
	    o So from all fours we'll step back
	        ▪ **[Demonstrate side-on]**
	        ▪ Keep your hips low
	        ▪ Low belly firm
	        ▪ Face parallel to the floor
	        ▪ Shoulder draw down the back
	        ▪ Push out through the heels and
	        ▪ Pull the chest forward
	           - Bend your knees to the mat to exit
	• Let's try that together, come onto all fours
	
	Hands and Arms
	• What we do with our hands is also important as it will effect how we use our shoulder muscles
	    o Make sure your middle finger points straight ahead and
	    o That your fingers are spread wide
	    o As with your feet, distribute your weight evenly to the base of each finger, your thumb and the heel of your hands
	    o **[Demonstrate face-on]**
	    o Now check your elbows
	    o The creases on the inside of your elbows we'll call the 'eyes' of your elbow – these need to be looking at each other
	        ▪ So let's put that all together

Do With / Watch Them	**From all-fours position – hold Rod for a few breaths**
	• Position your shoulders over your wrists
	• Now exhale and step the right foot back as far as you can
	• Step the left foot back
	• Keep breathing and
	    o Hold low belly firm
	    o Push out through the heels

	<ul><li>○ Strong arms</li><li>○ Draw the chest forward</li><li>○ Face parallel to the floor</li></ul><ul><li>Exhale, come to your knees</li></ul>
Introduction & Demonstration side-on *Pancha* **(Upward Dog)**	<ul><li>The next posture we'll learn is Upward Facing Dog</li></ul>**Enter Rod from all-fours**<ul><li>From our Rod</li><li>Inhaling, Upward Dog</li><li>Exhale, roll back, buttocks high</li></ul><ul><li>Upward Dog is a complex posture so we'll break it down into what we do with our legs, what we need do with our arms and then the head position</li></ul>
Workshop *Pancha* **(Upward Dog)** **Demonstration side-on**	**NOTE:** All of these, except 'Traction', are best workshopped in the 1st class **Strong Legs** <ul><li>The legs need to work strongly to support our low back</li><li>So first off lie on your belly<ul><li>○ Hands under your forehead</li><li>○ Feet hip-width apart</li></ul></li><li>Lift your kneecaps until your legs become so strong that your knees completely clear the floor</li><li>Now also press the top of your feet into the floor to work your legs more strongly<ul><li>○ Let's try all that together</li></ul></li></ul> **Arms Pull Forward** <ul><li>Position the elbows under your shoulders<ul><li>○ Come up onto your forearms*</li></ul></li><li>Again lift the kneecaps and press the top of your feet into the floor and</li><li>Inhaling, ground your hands and use your arms to pull the chest forward<ul><li>○ Let's do that together</li></ul></li></ul> **Traction** <ul><li>The idea in Upward Dog is to traction/lengthen the spine *From position above<ul><li>○ Strong legs</li><li>○ Press the top of your feet into the mat – these act as brakes and</li><li>○ Inhaling, pull your chest forward between your elbows</li></ul></li></ul> **Roll Over the Toes** <ul><li>Now let's revise how to transit from Rod into Upward Dog</li><li>Watch my feet</li></ul>

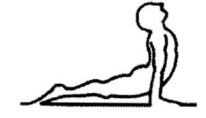

From Rod
- Inhaling, we roll over the toes
  - Until the feet point away
  - Front of the foot is on the mat
    - It's a great exercise to maintain the flexibility in your toes which is so important for walking
      - If you have a problem rolling all the way over your toes, try starting to roll over the toes and then step them over
- It is important that your Rod is long enough or you'll find you don't have enough space to roll forward
- Really pushing out through the heels will help you gain some extra space

- From all-fours position, straighten one leg out
  - Lets all try rolling over with one foot only
  - Now the other
  - And both feet together

NOTE:
- Stiffer students may need have their hands forward of their shoulders to be able to roll into Upward Dog

Roll Back
- To come out of Upward Dog, roll back over your toes, lift from your belly and take your buttocks high into the air
  - Imagine being lifted from your navel
- Now come down to your knees

Neck Position
- If you have or have had neck problems keep your head upright and look straight ahead
- Otherwise, lead with the chin to take your head back
- I'll show you
- **[Demonstrate - side on]**

- Let's put the whole thing together from our Rod
  - Remember: strong legs, arms pull you through, if you don't have a neck problem take your head back

---

Rod & Upward Dog

Do With / Watch Them

From all-fours position – hold for a few breaths
- Position your shoulders over your wrists
- Exhale step the right foot back as far as you can
- Step the left foot back
  - Push out through the heels
- Inhale roll over your toes
  - Keep breathing
  - Lift the kneecaps, press the feet into the mat
  - Pull the chest forward
  - Lead with the chin to take your head back
- Exhale, lift your buttocks up into the air, knees down to the floor, buttocks back to your heels (Child Posture)

Introduction & Demonstration side-on *Shat* (Downward dog) **Workshop Demonstration face-on**	• The last new posture of the sequence is called Downward Facing Dog
	• Unlike the other positions, we'll be holding this posture for 5 breaths
	• It looks like this
	
	From all-fours
	    ○ Exhale, straight, long Rod
	    ○ Inhale, roll over the toes into Upward Dog
	    ○ Exhale, buttocks high into Downward Dog
	    ○ 5 breaths here
	    ○ And exhaling, come down to your knees
	
	Puppy Posture
	• But before you can play dog, you have to be a 'puppy'
	• This preparation enables us to get the correct action at our shoulders before we take the weight into our hands
	• Watch me first
	• From where we were with our buttocks on our heels and our arms stretched out in front
	    ○ Work your arms back into your shoulders
	    ○ **[Exaggerate demonstration]**
	    ○ The shoulder blades draw down the back
	    ○ Chin down, back of the neck long
	    ○ Extend the top of your head forward toward your thumbs
	• Keep this action in your arms
	• Now tuck the toes under and straighten your legs
	    ○ Head down, buttocks up
	    ○ Feet straight and hip width apart
	• Let's try that together

Rod → Downward Dog **Do With / Watch Them**	**Add on from Rod**
	• Now let's add that on from the Rod
	
	From all-fours
	• Shoulders over the wrists
	• Exhale, step back into a long, straight Rod
	    ○ Push out through the heels
	• Inhale, roll over the toes into Upward Dog
	    ○ Pull the heart forward, brake with your feet
	• Exhale, buttocks high into Downward Dog
	    ○ Adjust your stance
	    ○ We work Downward Dog for 5 full breaths
	        ▪ Release your heels toward the floor
	        ▪ Feet hip-width apart, strong legs
	        ▪ Strong arms work back into the shoulders
	        ▪ Tuck your lowest ribs in towards your belly
	        ▪ Long neck, top of the head toward the thumbs
	• Exhale, come down to your knees

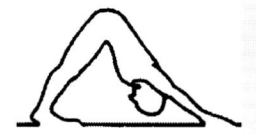

Workshop Downward Dog	**Stance**
	- If you have your feet too far from your hands the posture will be harder to hold
	  o You then need step your feet up a little
	- However, if your feet are too close to your hands, the posture will also become more difficult
	  o To find the stance that is right for you, enter Downward Dog from the Puppy. Memorise this distance and how it feels so you can adjust your feet to this each time you enter Downward Dog
	
	NOTE:
	- Entering Downward Dog from the Puppy will give students the ideal length of their stance – get them to make a mental note of how it looks and feels.
	
	Old Dog
	- Sadly, just as there are puppies, there are also old dogs
	- Initially, you may need to bend your knees in Downward Dog
	  o The good news is that eventually you will transform into a younger, more flexible dog!
	- From Downward Dog
	- Bend your knees and take the weight back into your feet and away from your hands [their buttocks should move back toward their feet]
	- Now work towards straightening your legs
	  o If straightening your legs moves the weight back into your hands you need to keep your knees bent

Samasthiti → **Downward Dog**
 	
Demonstrate side-on
 	
Do With / Watch Them
	- Let's take that from the top
	
	- **[Demonstrate from *Samasthiti* to Downward Dog]**
	
	- Let's do that together/ let me see you do it
	- Come to the top of your mat and stand in *Samasthiti*
	- Standing tall, feet ground evenly, heart lifted, spread your awareness over the whole of your body and breathe fully
	- Inhale, arms up, shoulders down, lift your chin, look to your thumbs
	- Exhale unlock your knees, fold forward, drop your head
	- Inhale lift your heart, shoulders above the wrists
	- Exhale, step back as far as you can to a long, strong, straight Rod
	  o Push out through the heels
	- Inhale, roll over the toes into Upward Dog
	  o Pull the heart forward, brake with your feet
	- Exhale, buttocks high into Downward Dog
	  o Adjust your stance
	  o We work Downward Dog for 5 full breaths
	    - Keep your feet active, your legs strong
	    - Actively tilt your pelvis forward at the hips
	    - Draw your lowest ribs away from your hands
	    - Shoulders broad and far away from the ears
	    - At the end of this exhalation, bend your knees, look between your thumbs
	- Exhale, come down to your knees

Introduction & Demonstration side-on *Sapta, Ashtau, Nava & Samasthiti*	**Exit**
	• That only leaves the exit back to *Samasthiti*
	• To do that we just reverse our first steps
	• I'll show you how
	    o Inhale, step your feet up, look up
	    o Exhale, fold forward [knees bent]
	    o Inhale come up, arms up
	    o Exhale, *Samasthiti*
	
	• If you can't make the step up in one single step take an extra one or two until your feet reach the level of your hands
	    o Let's do that together

Do With / Watch Them	• From Downward Dog
	    o Inhale, step or walk your feet up, lift your heart, look up
	    o Exhale, fold forward, thighs on your abdomen
	    o Inhale lift your head, come to upright, arms up
	    o Exhale, lower your arms and gaze to *Samasthiti*

Demonstration side-on Complete *Surya Namaskara A*	• That's the whole sequence. I'll put it together for you so you can see what it looks like
	    o Inhale, arms up, look up
	    o Exhale, bend forward
	    o Inhale, lift the heart
	    o Exhale, step back to Rod
	    o Inhale, Upward-facing Dog
	    o Exhale, Downward-facing Dog
	        ▪ 5 breaths here
	    o Inhale, step up and lift
	    o Exhale, forward
	    o Inhale, come up, arms up
	    o Exhale, *Samasthiti*

Do With / Watch Them	o [See Week 6 script for variations on detailed talk-through instructions of a complete *Surya Namaskara A*] ▪ [Repeat 3 times]

Padangushtasana   *drishti*: nose

Overview	- **Introduction *Padangustasana* and *Pada Hastasana***
	 - **Demonstrate**
	 - **Watch them do it**
	
	 NOTE:
	 - Step feet to hip width
	 - If 'straight feet' has not yet been taught, teach it here
	 - Demonstrate both postures at the same time
	     o You may show the hand grip before going forward
	 - Skip the step of doing the posture with them
	     o This is a simple posture and very similar to *Dve* and
	     o Student's hamstrings are usually quite sensitive by this stage
	 - Do not include *drishti* until after it is explained (week 3)

Introduction & Demonstration side-on *Padangustasana* *Pada Hastasana*	- We're going to do learn our first two standing postures - We enter it and each of our standing postures by bringing our hands into the symbolic gesture of a greeting, called *Namaste*, or a prayer position o **[Demonstrate]** - Watch me first From *Samasthiti* - Inhale hands in *Namaste* - Exhale feet hip-width apart - Inhale lift your heart - Exhale, fold forward [bent knees] - Inhale pick up the big toes and lift - Exhale forward for 5 breaths - Inhale lift the chest - Exhale change the hands to stand on your fingers - Inhale lift - Exhale forward again for 5 breaths - Inhale lift - Exhale, hands to the hips - Inhale come up - Exhale, *Samasthiti*
Padangustasana **Do With / Watch Them**	From *Samasthiti* - Inhale draw your hands up into *Namaste*, the greeting position - Exhale bend your knees and step your feet to land hip-width apart o Hands to your hips - Look down to your feet and imagine a line drawn from your second toe (the one alongside your big toe) through to the centre of your heel

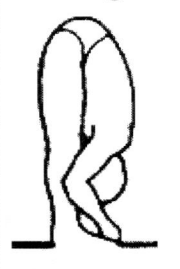

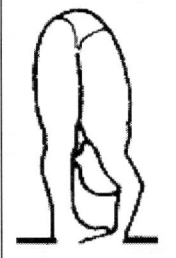

	<ul><li>○ This is the 'straight line' of your foot – now check that your feet are parallel to each other and straight</li><li>For all you cooks out there, our hand grasp is like taking a pinch of salt – first two fingers and thumb come together</li><li>Inhale ground your feet and lift up out of your hips</li><li>Exhale, strong legs, fold forward, abdomen on thighs</li><li>Inhale pick up your big toes and lift your heart</li><li>Exhale drop your head and fold forward<ul><li>○ Check that the four corners of your feet ground evenly and your insteps lift away from the floor</li><li>○ Lift your kneecaps and keep the legs working strongly</li><li>○ Keep your low abdomen close to your thighs and work towards straightening the legs a little more</li><li>○ Your shoulders draw away from your ears, your neck and spine relaxed and long</li><li>○ Continue to breath into the front, side, back and top of the chest, listening to the *ujjayi* sound</li></ul></li><li>Inhale lift your heart</li></ul>
Pada Hastasana Do With / Watch Them	<ul><li>Exhale place your fingers under your feet</li><li>Inhale lift your heart and</li><li>Exhale fold forward again<ul><li>○ 5 breaths here, breathing fully into all four corners of your chest</li><li>○ As you lift your shoulders away from the floor, let the weight of your head traction/lengthen your spine</li><li>○ The legs work strongly, the back releases<ul><li>▪ Imagine you're a drunk hanging over a fence - your legs become the fence, strong and supportive</li><li>▪ The whole of your back and spine lengthen and relax</li></ul></li></ul></li><li>Inhale lift your heart, your head and gaze</li><li>Exhale, stay forward/there, hands to your hips</li><li>Inhale come up to standing</li><li>Exhale, step or hop back to *Samasthiti*</li></ul>

Breath Meditation	*drishti*: **nose**
Overview	<ul><li>**Introduce the finishing postures and breathing meditation**</li><li>**Teach 'Open Cross-legged' sitting position**</li><li>**Demonstrate, do it with them and watch them do it**<ul><li>○ Approximately 10 rounds of breath</li></ul></li></ul>**NOTE:**<ul><li>Once you have instructed the sitting position, walk around to check they are doing it correctly</li><li>You can sit or walk around them to lead them through the breath meditation</li><li>Watch the height of their knees/curve in their low back and give extra blankets as needed</li><li>Eyes closed until they learn about drishti</li></ul>

	- Guide with instructions for at least 7 of 10 breaths
	  - Make your instructions logical (one leading to the next)
	  - You may also juxtapose instructions, eg: ground your sit-bones and lift your heart, etc
	  - It helps students to give instructions that are often lost with that phase of breath, eg: lengthen the spine w/ exhaling

Introduction & Demonstration	- In Ashtanga Yoga we start each class with a warm-up series which includes our sun salutations and a series of standing postures and then we'll finish each class with a series of finishing postures
	- These will include a breath meditation which we'll learn tonight
	- Everyone sitting on your blanket as we did earlier
	  - Check that your sit-bones (the bony prominences under your buttocks) are on the blanket, your feet and knees off the blanket
	  - If your knees are more than 10cm off the floor add another blanket
	    - This is important to keep the curve in your low back
	  - Open your cross-legged position by moving your heels away from your groins
	    - Your shins will form a straight line out in front of you
	    - Your ankles should be approximately under your knees
	  - Rest your hands, palms upward, upon your thighs
	  - Sit up tall and get comfortable
	  - We're going to be breathing together, try to keep pace with me
	    - Everyone exhale together

Do With / Watch Them	- Inhaling, release your sit-bones down into the blanket - Exhaling, lengthen through your spine and neck - Inhale, breath into the four areas of your chest - Exhale and keep your heart lifted and open - Inhale, draw your shoulders down away from your ears - Exhale drop your chin, soften your face - Inhale keep your legs relaxed, your low belly firm - Exhale the crown of your head rises toward the ceiling - Inhaling, listen to the sound of your breath - Exhaling, smooth and long, out through the nose - Inhale, feel your breath, warm and soothing as it enters - Exhale, allow the vitality of your breath to linger - Inhale feel the energy of the breath spreading over your torso and into your arms - Exhale, keep the breath smooth and long without straining - Inhale feel the life energy of your breath in your abdomen and legs - Exhale, lengthen your spine and neck, your face smooth and relaxed - Inhale let the expanse of the breath wash over your thoughts - Exhale clear your mind, follow your breathing - Inhale, long, smooth, soothing your mind - Exhale, through the nose, release any thoughts or tension - Inhale, feel your rib-cage expanding - Exhale, let the heart area float as your shoulders descend - Inhale, let the lungs fill, do not sucking the air in - Exhale, control the breath on the way out, long and smooth

	- Inhale, feel your chest expand in all directions
- Exhale, feel the lowest ribs draw back in toward the chest
- Inhale, allow the breath to wash over your thoughts
- Exhale, relax your mind, release the tendency to think
- Inhale, follow your breath, listen to its sound
- Exhale, let go to the rhythm of your breath
- Inhale feel how effortlessly the breath enters
- Exhale, smooth and slow and complete your exhalation
- Inhale let your ribs freely move, feel the lungs fill with prana
- Exhale, feel the chest deflate and the vitality the breath leaves
- Inhale feel yourself being breathed
- Exhale feel the gift of life the breath brings
- Inhale.... two.... three.... four....
- Exhale... two.... three.... four....
- Inhale ....
- Exhale ....

Shavasana

Overview	- **Introduce *Shavasana***
- **Demonstrate**
- **Teach students how to relax their bodies and their minds**

NOTE:
- Offer students an eye pillow
- The first two or three classes need a detailed *Shavasana* that comprehensively covers relaxing the physical body
- As the course progresses your may give less instructions
  - Make your instructions logical (one leading to the next)
- Once you have students relaxed do not move, shuffle papers or make any noise – be still and quiet yourself
- Adjust your tone and pace to induce a state of relaxation
- Taper off your instruction, making it clear that you are finished
- Be sure to vary your words: relax, soften, release, let go, etc
- Get students out of relaxation with a quiet, slow voice or use the chimes appropriately
- At the end remember to remind students to fold and stack their blankets neatly back in the pile |
| **Introduction & Demonstration** | - We'll finish every class with a relaxation exercise
- For your body to be healthy, it is not only important that our muscles are able to relax when we stop working them, but it is also important that we can slow our thoughts and pacify our mind
  - This is the original and main purpose of yoga
- This is the hardest posture you'll ever do perfectly
  - **[Demonstrate]**
- Actually, it is true. It may or may not be hard for you to relax your body but it is often difficult to slow down and relax our mind |

	- This posture is called *Shavasana*, which means 'corpse posture'
	  - So it's like playing dead
	  - It sounds a bit morbid but it is about learning to let go and dying is perhaps the biggest, and certainly final, exercise in letting go that each one of us will inevitably face
	- Once you are comfortable, try to lie still and not adjust your posture or fidget
	- I'll let you know when it's time to get up

	- Make sure that you are going to remain warm, you can use a blanket to cover you or also as a pillow
	- Lie on your back and bend up your knees if that's more comfortable
	  - If your knees are bent, place a rolled towel beneath your knees, separate your feet and let your knees come together to rest against each other
	  - If your legs are straight, let your feet roll open, as you relax your legs
	- Gently rock your head from side to side and relax your neck
	- Take your arms a little away from your sided and turn your palms upward
	- Gently close your eyes
	- Take a big breath in and let all your breath out in a big sigh [optional]
	  - Aaahhhhhh [Repeat a few times with them]
	- Make yourself as comfortable as possible and remain in this position unless you begin to experience real discomfort
	- Now completely let go of any control of your breath, let it fall to normal
	- Bring your awareness to your feet and check that they are relaxed, every joint in your feet and ankles, soft and relaxed
	- Feel where the back of your legs touch the mat and let them fall heavy and relaxed onto the mat
	- Relax your calf muscles and the muscles in the backs of your thighs
	- Soften your knee joints and feel the muscles in the front of your thighs release
	- Soften your hips, your groins and your buttocks
	- Feels your buttock muscles heavy and soft on the mat
	- Bring your awareness into the muscles along your spine and allow them to let go completely now that you've stopped working
	- Imagine each small joint of your vertebrae release any tension
	- Feel your abdomen soft and relaxed and notice your belly as it gently rises and falls with your breath
	- Feel the gentle movement of your ribs as your breath becomes shorter and shallow
	- Let the front of your throat be soft, the back of your neck relaxed
	- Release any tension from your head and face
	- Relax your shoulders, let them fall heavy toward the floor
	- Bring your awareness into your elbow joints and your wrists and let them soften as they release
	- Notice the fingers of your hands curl as the hands relax
	- Let your whole body be soft, heavy and easy. Let it feel like you're melting into the earth below.

- Let the skin on the whole of your body and face feel smooth
- With your whole body relaxed, draw your awareness away from your physical body and become aware of your thoughts.
- Without trying to change anything, watch your thoughts as they come and go
- See them as if they were clouds against a deep blue sky
- As each thought comes along, watch it and let it go on past
- Don't allow yourself to get hooked into one particular thought but watch it arise, watch it pass, and let it go
- Begin to focus on the deep blue sky beyond your thoughts and allow yourself to relax
- Notice that as you relax, that expanse of deep, open space also expands and eventually your mind will fall still
- Enjoy this quiet, still space and allow yourself to truly rest

- **[CHIMES or CHANT or]**
- Gently bring your awareness back into the room
- Slowly bring your awareness back into your body
- Begin to move your fingers and toes
- When you're ready, bend up your knees and roll over onto one side
- Rest there for a moment
- Then slowly and in your own time come up to sitting

Week 2

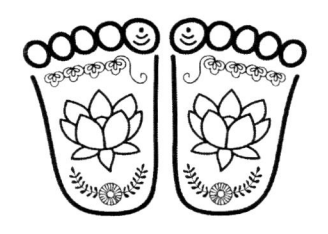

WEEK 2 • The Energy System

Class Overview	• Greeting, revision last class, introduction of today's class • Revise breathing exercise • Revise *Ujjayi Pranayama* • Introduce & teach the *bandhas* • Revise *Samasthiti* with *bandhas* • Revise *Surya Namaskara A* • Teach *Surya Namaskara B* • Revise or Teach *Padangustasana & Pada Hastasana* • Teach *Trikonasana* • Teach *Yogamudrasana* • Teach *Jnana mudra* with breath mediation • Teach *Uttpluthi* • *Shavasana* NOTE: • Incorporate the *ujjayi pranayama* and a description of the *bandhas* in *Samasthiti* and every new posture • Hand out sun salutation sheet

REVISION: Breathing Exercise

Introduction	• Good morning/hello everyone. How have you gone doing your sun salutations every day and practising your breathing? • Last week we learnt how to breath fully using our diaphragm muscle so for all of you who haven't been practising, let's revise that now before we start with our postures. ○ Everyone lie on your back and bend up your knees

Watch Them	• **See Week 1 script**
	    ○ Go straight into exercise without 'normal breathing'
	    ○ Come back up to sitting on your blankets
	        • Are there any questions on that?

Bandhas	

Overview	• **Introduce the *bandhas***
	  ○ **Energetic application/benefits**
	  ○ **Physical application/benefits**
	    ▪ Incorporate a description of the *bandhas* in each posture

Introduction & Exercise	• So we've learnt how to breath fully and last week we also learnt how to direct the breath by narrowing the passage of the breath or the *glottis*.
	  ○ This made the characteristic sound of our *ujjayi* breath system
	  ○ Do you all remember how to make the sound?
	    ▪ Let's all do the sound together
	      - **[Demonstrate sound]**
	  ○ This type of breathing - *Ujjayi pranayama* – really helps to heat up the body and is one of the reasons people gain flexibility quickly when practising *Ashtanga Yoga*
	
	• Last week we also talked about the concept of *pranayama*, where the breath is recognised as life force.
	  ○ This life force permeates the whole of our body but accumulates in various channels within the body.
	  ○ The main/major energy channel runs along the spine.
	    ▪ It's called the *sushumna* and is analogous to our spinal cord
	
	• Today we are going to learn a couple of locks to enable us to both contain and cultivate the energy within this central channel/vessel.
	  ○ The first lock is the root lock or *mulha bandha*
	    ▪ *Bandha* means lock and *mulha* means root
	    ▪ It's called the root lock because it is at the base or root of the *sushumna*/spine and
	    ▪ It helps seal energy in at the base of the *sushumna*/spine
	      - In yoga it is said that every posture grows up out of *mulha bandha* like a lotus flower
	  ○ Physically, to engage *mulha banda* we engage the pelvic floor
	    ▪ The pelvic floor is the muscular sling between your pubic bone and your tail bone
	    ▪ The action is a gentle lifting, sucking or contraction of this area
	      - Try that
	      - Gently contract the area between your pubic and tail bones until you feel a lifting sensation
	      - It is a similar sensation to stopping urination
	        ○ Could everyone feel that?
	  ○ The second lock or *bandha* is called *uddiyana bandha*
	    ▪ *Uddiyana* means flying upward
	    ▪ The energy in the central channel/*sushumna* tends to leak out and stagnate at its base
	    ▪ *Mulha bandha* contains the energy within the vessel/channel and *uddiyana bandha* helps to lift it up the spine

	<ul><li>○ *Uddiyana bandha* is engaged by contracting the lower abdomen or the *transverse abdominal* muscle<ul><li>▪ The transverse abdominal muscle wraps around the torso like a corset</li><li>▪ It is the deepest layer of your abdominal muscles and</li><li>▪ Is an important core stabilising muscle for your low back</li><li>▪ Uddiyana bandha is naturally engaged when you sneeze, cough or laugh</li><li>▪ Everyone place your hands just inside your hip bones on your lower abdomen<ul><li>- Now laugh<ul><li>• Can you feel the muscles contract/engage under your fingers?</li><li>• This is your transverse abdominal muscle bracing your lower abdomen</li><li>• So for the rest of today's class I want you to pretend that everything I say is completely hilarious, but being so polite, you only almost burst our laughing</li></ul></li></ul></li><li>▪ Be careful to only engage the lower part of your abdomen, below your navel so you do not restrict the action of your diaphragm<ul><li>• It's a bit like a cowboy with his belt around his hips, but his belly above the belt is somewhat relaxed</li></ul></li></ul></li><li>○ Attempt to engage *mulha and uddiyana bandha* both on your inhalation and your exhalation, that is, throughout the entire yoga practice</li></ul>
Watch Them	<ul><li>Sitting up tall on your blankets</li><li>Begin to breath fully into the four areas of your chest, the front, the sides, the back and up into the top lobes of your lungs</li><li>Smoothly exhale being sure to make the *ujjayi* sound as you breathe</li><li>Keep breathing fully and</li><li>Gently contract the pelvic floor, creating a lifting sensation at the base of the spine</li><li>Now brace your lower abdomen as if you were about to laugh and feel your lower belly become firm</li><li>Do a couple more rounds of breath, and then relax</li><li>Let's come to standing and apply that to our postures</li></ul>

REVISION: *Samasthiti*	
Watch Them	<ul><li>Remember our first posture is *Samashtiti,* the equal standing pose<ul><li>○ See Week 1 script</li></ul></li></ul>

REVISION: *Surya Namaskara A*	

Overview	• Being a revision of *Surya Namaskara A* the main difference will be that you can
	   o Leave out the middle step of doing the move with them
	   o Combine the first three moves (*ekam, dve, trini*) as the first demonstration and exercise
	• Otherwise breakdown *Surya Namaskara A* as you did in the first class
	   o This is necessary as they make not have done it since last class (weekly students) and/or you may have a student who missed class one
	   o Remember this is their first few times of doing *Surya Namaskara* – it will not be boring for them to break it down and it will help them to get it right
	• Workshop any areas from 'Synchronising Breath with Movement' or '*Surya Namaskara A*' that you did not get to workshop in week 1

Introduction & Demonstration	• Maintain *Samasthiti* and watch me as I demonstrate the sun salutation or *Surya Namaskara* that we learnt last week
Watch Them	• See Week 1 script o Lead them through four *Surya Namaskara A*

Surya Namaskara B	

Overview	• **Introduce *Surya Namaskara B***
	• **Teach *Utkatasana***
	   o Arms only
	   o Legs only
	      ▪ Workshop position of pelvis
	   o Arms & legs together
	
	NOTE:
	• Repeat each part at least three times to cover all necessary instructions
	• The arm action for the entrance and exit of *Surya Namaskara B* are different
	   o You may teach both at the beginning or otherwise teach the arm movement for exiting *Surya Namaskara B* at the end of the sun salutation

	- **Teach *Virabhadrasana***
	  o First from standing
	    ▪ Workshop knee position
	  o Then from Downward Dog
	    ▪ Workshop foot position
	    ▪ Workshop squaring the hips
	  o Then with a *Vinyasa* between sides
	
	- **Teach complete *Surya Namaskara B***
	
	NOTE:
	- For each part do: 'Demonstration', 'Do with them', 'Watch them'
	- Change the direction you are facing during the various demonstrations
	- Beginners can be given an extra breath to enter *Virabhadrasana*
	- Initially the step-up into *Virabhadrasana* is done at the end of the exhalation taken for Downward Dog
	- Workshop any part of the sun salutations not yet workshopped

Introduction	- So that is the A version of our sun salutation, now we're going to learn a B version - It uses a lot of the same movements with two new postures added o Let me show you the first one

Demonstrate face-on or side-on *Utkatasana* ARMS	**Arms**
	- We'll do the arms first
	  o Inhale arms up in front, look up
	  o Exhale down through the centre
	  o Back to *Samasthiti*
	    ▪ Let's do that together

Do With / Watch Them	- Inhale, palms together, bring the arms straight up in front, look to the thumbs - Exhale, lower your hands down through the centre, close to your heart - Again - Inhale, follow your thumbs with your gaze as you raise your arms - Exhale, lower the arms, down the centre, past your heart - Once more - Inhale, keep your arms straight as you raise them up, look up - Exhale, hands pass down past your heart centre

Demonstrate side-on & Workshop *Utkatasana* **LEGS**	**Legs**
	• This is what we do with the legs
	    o Inhaling, bend the knees deeply
	    o Exhaling, back to *Samasthiti*
	
	• Before you try that just take note of what happens with your low back
	    o We don't stick our buttocks out
	        ▪ [Demonstrate]
	    o And we don't tuck our tail under
	        ▪ [Demonstrate]
	    o Instead, keep the natural curve in your low back and simply bend your knees without changing the position of your pelvis
	        ▪ [Demonstrate]
	• Let's do that together

Do With / Watch Them	• Inhale, deeply bend your knees, keep the curve in your low back
	• Exhale, straighten your legs, *Samashtiti*
	    o Again
	• Inhale, drop your sit bones, weight in the heels/ the heels keep contact with the mat/ the heels stay grounded
	• Exhale, back up
	    o Once more
	• Inhale, squat low keep the knees together/touching
	• Exhale back up to *Samashtiti*

Demonstrate *Utkatasana*	**Arms & Legs Together**
	• So now we put them together
	    o Inhale arms up in front as we bend the knees
	    o Exhale hands down the centre, legs straighten
	    o Back to *Samashtiti*
	
	• This posture is called *Utkatasana*, the power pose
	    o *Utkatasana* develops a lot of power in the legs and buttocks
	        ▪ Let's try that together

Do With / Watch Them	• Inhale, drop your sit bones, palms together, arms straight up in front, gaze to your thumbs
	• Exhale, hands down past the heart centre, straighten your legs
	    o Again
	• Inhale, deeply bend your knees, shoulders down, raise your arms up in front, gaze up
	• Exhale, lower your hands down the midline, back to *Samashtiti*
	    o Once more
	• Inhale, squat low, shoulders heavy, straight arms, palms together, gaze follows your thumbs
	• Exhale, lower the arms close down through the centre, legs straighten

Introduce, Demonstrate & Workshop *Virabhadrasana* **From Standing**	- The second posture that makes the sun salutation B longer and more challenging is the warrior posture or *Virabhadrasana*
	  o We stand proud and strong like a warrior
	- Watch me first
	
	From Standing
	- Left foot at 45 degrees
	- Inhale, take a long step back
	- Exhale, hands to hips
	  o Square the shoulders, torso and hips to the front foot/front of your mat
	  o **[Demonstration: exaggerate movement]**
	- Inhale, arms up, gaze up
	- Exhale arms down
	- Inhale, step your back foot back up
	
	Knee Over Ankle
	- It is very important that you knee does not go beyond your ankle
	  o This means less weight is borne through the knee which protects your knee joint
	- You may need widen your stance
	  o Work toward having your thigh parallel to the floor with the knee above the ankle
	- Let's try that

Do With / Watch Them & Workshop	**From Standing**
	- Left foot at 45 degrees
	- Inhaling, take a long step back with the right foot
	- Exhale, hands to your hips
	  o Now check that your stance is wide enough that when you bend the front knee it does not travel beyond your ankle
	    ▪ Widen your stance if you need to
	- Inhale, raise the arms
	  o Exhale, arms down and step the back foot up to the front
	    ▪ Other side
	
	Degrees of Foot Position
	- To protect our knee joint we will often need to place the foot in a certain position
	- Look at my feet
	- **[Demonstrate each]**
	  o Let's call this position zero degrees (feet straight)
	  o This is then 45 degrees
	  o And this, 90 degrees
	- When we square our hips if we do not let the foot come with the hip, the knee will have to take up the rotation
	  o Having the toes point in the same direction as your knee removes any stress from the knee joint
	- With your right foot at 45 degrees
	- Inhale and take a long step forward with the left foot
	- Exhale, hands to your hips
	  o Again check that your stance is wide enough that your knee is positioned above your ankle
	    ▪ Widen your stance if you need to

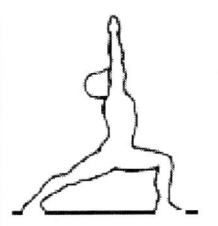

	Squaring the Hips
	• For most people it is almost impossible to square the hips 100%
	• You can, however, fully square your shoulders and torso and then square your hips as much as you can
	    o In *Virabhadrasana*, with your hands on your hips, look down to your hands - now work towards your hands being on the same level
	    o Work the back hip forward and the front hip back to level your hands and square your hips

Demonstrate *Virabhadrasana*
 	
From Downward Dog
	From Downward Dog
	• In the sun salutation, we actually enter *Virabhadrasana*, the warrior pose, from downward dog
	    o Let me show you
	• From Downward Dog
	    o Inhale, up on the toes, right foot steps up
	    o Exhale, come up, back foot grounded at 45 degrees
	    o Inhale, arms up
	    o Exhale, hands down and into rod
	    o Inhale, up dog
	    o Exhale, down dog
	        ▪ Left side
	    o Inhale, up on the toes, left foot up
	    o Exhale, come up, square the hips
	    o Inhale, arms up
	    o Exhale, down and back to rod
	    o Inhale, up dog
	    o Exhale, down dog
	        ▪ Come to your knees
	
	Extra Step-Up
	• Initially you may not be able to step-up far enough to be at a wide enough stance
	• Step-up as far as you can, come up and then take another step forward until your stance is wide enough
	    o Let's try that together
	
	NOTE:
	• When exiting *Virbhadrasana*, if the knee travels forward beyond the ankle, slide the back foot away into a deeper lunge

Do With / Watch Them	• As you exhale into Downward Dog
	    o Stay up on your toes and step the right foot up between your hands
	    o Inhale, come up, plant your back foot at 45 degrees
	        ▪ Widen your stance now if you need to
	    o Exhale, hands to your hips, square them
	    o Inhale, raise the arms, look to your thumbs
	    o Exhale hand down either side of the right foot step back to rod
	    o Inhale, updog, strong legs
	    o Exhale, buttocks high into down dog

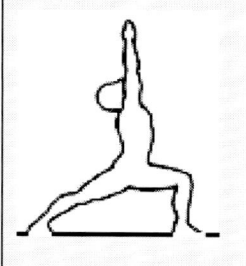

	- Left side
	    - Inhale, on your toes, step the left foot up
	    - Exhale, back heel down, square your hips
	    - Inhale, arms up, look up
	    - Exhale, hands down and back into a rod
	    - Inhale, up dog, pull your chest through
	    - Exhale, push off your hands into down dog
	        - Come to your knees

Demonstrate *Surya Namaskara B*	- Ok, I'll put the whole thing together, *Surya Namaskara B*
	    - Inhale, deep squat, arms up
	    - Exhale, fold forward
	    - Inhale lift, look up
	    - Exhale, step back to rod
	    - Inhale, Upward Dog
	    - Exhale, step the right foot up
	    - Inhale, come up
	    - Exhale, squaring off
	    - Inhale, arms up, look up
	    - Exhale, back to rod
	    - Inhale, updog
	    - Exhale, downdog, left foot up
	    - Inhale, back foot 45 degrees
	    - Exhale, square off
	    - Inhale, arms up, *Virabhadrasana*
	    - Exhale, rod
	    - Inhale, updog
	    - Exhale, downdog
	        - 5 breaths in Downward Dog
	    - Inhale, step the feet up
	    - Exhale, fold forward
	    - Inhale, a deep *Utkatasana*
	    - Exhale arms down, *Samasthiti*

Do With / Watch Them	[Choose from the instructions listed]
Samasthiti	• In *Samasthiti*, ground the four corners of your feet, lift the insteps • Grow your legs tall and strong • Continue a sensation of lifting from you feet, up your legs and into your pelvis, feeling the lift of your pelvic floor, which is *mulha bandha* • Let your sit bones feel heavy, keep the buttocks firm but not clenched • Lightly brace your lower abdomen, engaging *uddiyana bandha* • Lift your heart, open the back of your chest and breathe in all directions, feel your ribs move/float as you breathe • Loop your shoulders back and down, keeping the shoulder blades broad on your back • Lightly extend through your arms and fingers • Lengthen your neck, shoulders & ears backing away from each other • Gently draw your ears back in line with your shoulders • Drop the chin slightly to soften your throat/front of your neck • Soften your face and gaze softly out in front of you • Check that your posture feels light and balanced • Tune into the sound of your breath o Ready for *Surya Namaskara B*, everyone exhale together
Ekam 1	• Inhale, drop your sit bones, knees together, arm straight up in front, gaze to your thumbs • Inhale, deeply bend your knees, shoulders down raise your arms out in front, gaze up • Inhale, squat low, shoulders heavy, straight arms, palms together, follow your thumbs • Inhale, as you lower your buttocks, raise your arms, lift your gaze to follow your thumbs • Inhale, drop the buttocks, shoulders down, arms up in front, gaze to your thumbs
Dve 2	• Exhale, hands down past your heart centre, drop your head • Exhale, hands down the centre, strong legs, belly touches the thighs • Exhale, fold forward, splay your sit bones, belly kissing the thighs • Exhale, hands down, low belly firm, fold forward, drop your head • Exhale, take the long way down, fold at the hips, drop your head • Exhale, strong legs, fold forward, work to keep the curve in your low back
Trini 3	• Inhale, fingers touch the floor, lift your heart, your head and your gaze • Inhale, lift your chest, shoulders down, back of the neck long • Inhale, lift your chest, broaden your shoulders, look up • Inhale, lift your heart, widen your collarbones, look up • Inhale, heart, head and gaze lift, shoulders down • Inhale lift your heart, your head and your gave, shoulders broad

Chatvari 4	• Exhale, step back into the rod, low belly strong • Exhale, fingers spread wide, weight in the hands, step back • Exhale, back into rod, push out through the heels • Exhale, rod, draw the chest forward between your hands • Exhale, rod, push out through the heels, pull your heart forward • Exhale, rod, pinch your shoulder blades together on your back • Exhale, rod, drop your chin, face parallel to the floor • Exhale step back to rod, long, strong and straight
Pancha 5	• Inhale, roll over your toes to updog, draw your chest forward • Inhale to Upward Dog, use your arms to draw you forward • Inhale, Upward Dog, strong legs, draw the heart forward, look up • Inhale, strong legs, brace your low belly, lift the chin, look up • Inhale, press the top of your feet into the mat, gaze upward • Inhale, spread the fingers, roll the shoulder back and down • Inhale, use you feet as brakes, the arms to traction your spine
Shat 6	• Exhaling downdog, stay up on your toes
Sapta 7	• Step the right foot up – take an extra step here if needed • Inhaling ground the back foot, 45 degrees, come upright • Exhale hands to your hips, square them • Inhale, raise the arms, shoulders down, gaze to your thumbs
Ashtau 8	• Exhale, hands down, step back to rod • Exhale down, back to rod, push out through your heels • Exhale down, back to rod, pull your sternum/chest forward • Exhale, rod, shoulder blades together
Nava 9	• Inhale roll over your toes to Upward Dog, strong legs • Inhale, updog, pull the chest forward • Inhale, updog, brake with your feet, pull your heart through • Inhale updog, strong legs, lift the kneecaps • Inhale, updog, shoulders back and down
Dasha 10	• Exhaling buttocks up to downdog, up on your toes • Exhaling, push off your hands into downdog, up on your toes • Exhaling, push the buttocks high into downdog, up on your toes • Exhaling buttocks high into downdog, up on your toes

Ekadasha 11	- Step the right foot up to your hands - Inhaling ground the back foot 45 degrees, come up hands to your hips - Exhale, square your hips to the front foot - Inhale, arms up, shoulders down, chin up to gaze to your thumbs
Dvadasha 12	- Exhale, hands down, step back to rod - Exhale down, back to rod, push out through your heels - Exhale down, back to rod, pull your sternum/chest forward - Exhale, rod, shoulder blades together
Trayodasha 13	- Inhale roll over your toes to Upward Dog, strong legs - Inhale, updog, pull the chest forward - Inhale, updog, brake with your feet, pull your heart through - Inhale, updog, pull the chest through - Inhale updog, strong legs, lift the kneecaps - Inhale, updog, shoulders back and down

Chaturdasha 14	- Exhale, push off your hands, buttocks high into downward dog
	- Exhale, buttocks high into Downward Dog
	- Exhale, butt up, head down, Downward Dog
	  - Drop your heels, check your feet are straight and hip-width apart
	  - Heavy heels, strong legs, gaze between your knees
	  - Splay your sit bones wide and work them to the ceiling
	  - Tip the pelvis forward, try to recreate the curve in your low back
	  - Draw up from the centre of your pelvic floor, engaging *mulha bandha*
	  - Keep the lowest part of you abdomen firm with *uddiyana bandha*
	  - Elongate the whole of your spine, including your neck
	  - Use the weight of your head to lengthen your neck
	  - Back of the head in line with the rest of your spine
	  - Drop your chin to keep the front of the neck soft
	  - Soften the lowest ribs back into your abdomen
	  - Draw your shoulder blades back up toward the hips
	  - Breathe into the space between your shoulder blades
	  - Keep the shoulder blades broad on your back
	  - Feel the arms working back into your shoulder joints
	  - Strong arms, feel them propping you up
	  - Work your shoulders down away from your ears
	  - Crown of the head works forward towards your thumbs
	  - Spread your fingers, middle finger points straight ahead
	  - Check that the base of your fingers and thumb touch the mat
	  - Ground down from the base of the little finger to the base of the thumb and gently push the mat away with your hands
	  - Ground your hands, transfer your weight back toward your feet
	  - If your knees are bent, gently work toward straightening them
	  - Soften your face and gaze softly between your knees
	  - Breathe fully, feel your ribs move with the breath
	  - Breathe into the front, sides and back of your chest
	  - Feel your ribs float as you breathe
	  - Listen to the sound of your breath

	<ul><li>Heels heavy, strong legs, hands grounding, strong arms</li><li>Imagine you're a tent, your hands and feet the pegs grounding, your hips the highest point</li><li>Feel the strength and support of your limbs as you elongate your spine</li><li>Strong arms and legs, relax and release your spine</li><li>At the end of your exhalation, bend your knees, look to your thumbs</li></ul>
Panchadasa 15	<ul><li>Inhale, step your feet up, lift your heart, head and gaze</li><li>Inhale pull the feet up between your hands, look up</li><li>Inhale, use your arms to step up, keep lifting, look up</li><li>Inhale, keep the buttocks high as you step the feet up</li></ul>
Shodasha 16	<ul><li>Exhale, fold forward, splay your sit bones, belly kissing the thighs</li><li>Exhale, fold forward, work towards straightening the legs</li><li>Exhale, forward, low belly firm, drop your head</li><li>Exhale, forward, strong legs, long spine and neck</li></ul>
Saptadasha 17	<ul><li>Inhale, drop your sit bones, knees together, arm straight up in front, gaze to your thumbs</li><li>Inhale, deeply bend your knees, shoulders down, raise your arms out in front, gaze up</li><li>Inhale, squat low, shoulders heavy, straight arms, palms together, follow your thumbs</li><li>Inhale, as you lower your buttocks, raise your arms, lift your gaze to follow your thumbs</li><li>Inhale, drop the buttocks, shoulders down, arms up in front, gaze to your thumbs</li></ul>
Samasthiti	<ul><li>Exhale, arms down back to *Samasthiti*</li><li>Exhale, arms down, legs straight, *Samasthiti*</li><li>Exhale, lower your arms, straighten your legs, *Samasthiti*</li><li>Exhale, *Samasthiti*, the equal-standing pose</li><li>Exhale, *Samasthiti*, gaze softly down</li></ul>

REVISION: *Padangustasana & Pada Hastasana*

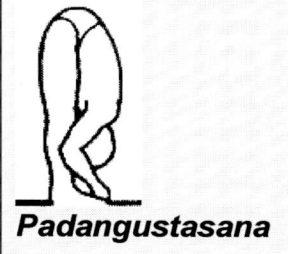

Padangustasana	• Let's do the first of the standing postures we learnt last week
	• Do you remember them?
	• I'll show you to refresh your memory…
	    ○ **[Demonstrate both postures]**
	• Let me see you do it
	    ○ **[Watch them]**
	• From *Samasthiti*
	• Inhale draw your hands up into *Namaste*
	• Exhale bend your knees and step your feet hip-width apart
	    ○ Hands to your hips
	• Inhale ground your feet and lift up out of your hips
	• Exhale, strong legs, fold forward, bend your knees
	• Inhale pick up your big toes and look up
	• Exhale drop your head, shoulders lift away from the floor
	    ○ Continue to breath into the front, side, back and top of the chest, listening to the *ujjayi* sound
	    ○ Check that the four corners of your feet ground evenly and your insteps lift away from the floor
	    ○ Continue to lift your pelvic floor and lightly brace the lower abdomen
	    ○ Keep your low abdomen close to your thighs and work towards straightening the legs a little more
	    ○ Your shoulder draw away from your ears, your neck and spine extending long
	• Inhale lift your heart

Pada Hastasana	• Exhale place your fingers under your feet and fold forward again
	    ○ Breath fully, feel your rib cage move and listen to the sound of your breath
	    ○ As you lift your shoulders away from the floor, let the weight of your head traction/lengthen your spine
	    ○ The legs work strongly, the back releases
	        ▪ Imagine you're hanging over a fence where your legs become the fence, strong and supportive
	        ▪ Allow the whole of your back and spine lengthen and relax
	• Inhale lift your heart, your head and your gaze
	• Exhale, stay forward/there, hands to your hips
	• Inhale come up to standing
	• Exhale, step back to *Samasthiti*

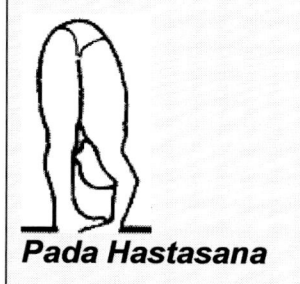

Trikonasana	drishti: thumb

Overview	<ul><li>**Introduce *Trikonasana***</li><li>**Demonstrate**</li><li>**Teach hip action separately**<ul><li>Workshop feet & stance</li><li>Workshop hip action</li></ul></li><li>**Teach complete *Trikonasana***<ul><li>Workshop staying on one plane</li><li>Do with them</li><li>Watch them</li></ul></li></ul>**NOTE:**<ul><li>Teach hip and trunk actions separately</li><li>Give the option to those with neck problems to keep their neck straight/head centre and to gaze straight ahead<ul><li>If this is still difficult they can gaze down to their foot</li></ul></li><li>Bring the gaze back to straight ahead to help students balance</li></ul>
Introduce & Demonstrate face-on *Trikonasana*	<ul><li>The next standing posture we'll learn looks like a triangle. For that reason it's *Sanskrit* name, *Trikonasana* means triangle posture<ul><li>Watch me first</li></ul></li><li>Inhale *Namaste*</li><li>Exhale step to the right, arms out shoulder height</li><li>Right foot opens 90 degrees, left foot in slightly</li><li>Drop the right hip</li><li>Inhale reach over the right foot</li><li>Exhale place the hand down, look up to the thumb<ul><li>5 breaths here</li></ul></li><li>Inhale look to the front, come up</li><li>Exhale change sides, left foot 90 degrees, right foot about 5 degrees</li><li>Inhale, reach out over the left foot</li><li>Exhale down and if steady, gaze up to the thumb<ul><li>5 breaths</li></ul></li><li>Inhale, gaze straight ahead and come up</li><li>Exhale, step back to *Samasthiti*</li></ul>
Workshop Feet & Stance	**Feet & Stance**<ul><li>OK, let's look at our feet and the length of our stance</li><li>Try to land with your feet straight/at 0 degrees. Adjust them as necessary</li><li>The width of your feet needs to be approximately one metre wide<ul><li>If your stance is too short or too long the pose will be much more difficult</li></ul></li><li>Now we position our feet for the right side. We do this by<ul><li>Opening the right foot to 90 degrees, the left foot turns in slightly<ul><li>The basic rule is that you foot will always point in the same direction as your knee</li></ul></li></ul></li></ul>

Workshop Hips	• This means there will be no rotation at your knee, which helps to protect the knee joint ○ Now check that your ankles remain in line with each other **Hip Action** • Ok now let's focus in on what you need to do with your hips • We tilt the hips/pelvis sideways ○ The right side of your pelvis drops, the left side tilts upward • To change sides, square off the feet • The left foot turns out 90 degrees, the right in slightly • Tilt the pelvis/hips down to the left ○ Let's try that together, we'll do both sides
Workshop Complete *Trikonasana*	• Now we'll add in the rest to make the posture, *Trikonasana* • Entering from *Samasthiti*, inhale hands into *Namaste* • Exhale step to the right, arms out shoulder height • Inhale adjust the feet for the right side/ ○ Right foot 90 degrees, left foot in slightly • Drop the right hip • Look to the right foot and inhaling, reach out over it • Exhale place the hand down ○ 5 breaths here • Inhale look to the front, come up **Working In One Plane** • When you reach out over the foot check that you do not lean forward • Attempt to stay on one plane – over the leg • Imagine that you are between two planes of glass ○ **[Demonstrate face-on]** • Exhale change sides ○ Left foot opens 90 degrees, right foot in about 5 degrees • Inhale, looking to the left foot, reach out over it • Exhale down and if steady, look up to the thumb ○ 5 breaths • Inhale look back to the front and come up • Exhale, step back to *Samasthiti* **Head & Neck** • If it is not comfortable for your neck to look up to the thumb, keep your head centred and instead look straight ahead • If that is still uncomfortable for you, look down to your foot
Do With / Watch Them	• *Samasthiti* • Inhale hands up to *Namaste* • Exhale step to your right, landing your feet about 1m wide, arms out shoulder height ○ Keep the arms up, hovering above your hips • Open your right foot to 90 degrees and turn your left foot in slightly • Inhale look to your right foot, and pretending you are between two planes of glass, reach out as far as you can

	<ul><li>Exhale place your hand down to your leg and if comfortable, look up to your left thumb, or gaze straight ahead<ul><li>Keep breathing, keeping your breath full and the chest moving</li><li>As your ground the feet, lift the insteps, lift your kneecaps</li><li>Check that your right knee is not locked out but rather just a fraction bent</li><li>Keep both shoulders down away from your ears</li><li>Lengthen the back of your neck</li></ul></li><li>Look back straight ahead and inhaling come up</li><li>Exhale change sides, left foot 90 degrees, right foot in about 5 degrees</li><li>Inhale, without leaning forward, extend out over the left foot OR</li><li>Keep your arms above your legs and reach as far as you can over your left foot</li><li>Exhale left shoulder over left leg, right shoulder above the left, gaze up to your thumb<ul><li>5 breaths, strong legs, keep the kneecaps lifted</li><li>Draw up from the pelvic floor using *mulha bandha*</li><li>Keep the lower abdomen firm as you engage *uddiyana bandha*</li><li>Check that your neck is in line with the rest of your spine</li><li>Lengthen your neck and spine as you draw your shoulders down</li></ul></li><li>Inhale gaze back to the front and come up</li><li>Exhale, step back to *Samasthiti*</li></ul>

Yoga Mudrasana   *drishti:* nose

Overview	<ul><li>**Introduce *Yoga Mudrasana***</li><li>**Demonstrate**</li><li>**Watch them**</li></ul>**NOTE:**<ul><li>Students must sit in an 'open' cross-legged position. Otherwise their sit bones will come off the floor and they will topple forward</li><li>For the same reason, students are not up on a blanket unless they are extremely stiff<ul><li>Extremely stiff students will also need to bring their arms forward of their torso</li></ul></li><li>You can go forward with students into the posture but then come up so they can hear your instructions</li><li>Do not incorporate the *drishti* until Week 3<ul><li>Students can close their eyes</li></ul></li></ul>
Introduce & Demonstrate face-on	<ul><li>Today we'll add in some additional finishing postures</li><li>As we did last week, we'll sit in an open cross-legged position<ul><li>This means moving your heels away from your groins<ul><li>The shins form a straight line out in front of you and</li><li>Your ankles will be approximately positioned under your knees</li></ul></li></ul></li></ul>

Yoga Mudrasana	• Our new posture is *Yoga Mudrasana* or the seal of *yoga*. In this pose we seal the energy or *prana*, that the practice cultivates, into the body
	   o We clasp the arms behind our back
	   o Inhale, lift out of the hips
	   o Exhale, fold forward
	
	   o [Come up]
	   o We'll hold the posture for up to 10 breaths
	     ▪ Let's try that

Do With / Watch Them	• Sitting in an open cross-legged position • Check that your ankles sit approximately beneath your knees • Now clasp your elbows behind your back • If you can't yet reach your elbows grasp your forearm • Inhale, lift out of the hips • Exhale, fold forward, just as far as you go • Relax your neck • Stay there and breath fully • Inhaling come back to sitting upright

Jnana Mudra   *drishti:* **nose**

Overview	▪ Introduce *Jnana Mudra* ▪ **Demonstrate** ▪ **Do it with them and/or watch them do it** **NOTE:** ▪ Students should sit up on a blanket – give extra blankets to those students whose knees are still >10cm above the floor ▪ Do this posture with them or watch them do it ▪ The *drishti* is taught and then incorporated in Week 3's class

Introduce & Demonstrate face-on
 	
Jnana Mudra
	• Firstly, sit up on your blanket
	   o Check that your sit-bones are on the blanket, feet off the blanket
	
	• In our next posture we'll also form a seal or *mudra* – it is a seal of intention.
	• We use our fingers symbolically to represent this seal
	   o Symbolically, each finger represents a different aspect of our being. For example, the pointing finger represents individual consciousness and the thumb represents universal consciousness. We join the two into what is called the seal of knowledge. This is the knowledge that we are one and a part of the universal whole – that each of us shares the same life-force, the one and same consciousness.

Do With / Watch Them	• Sitting upright, if you feel comfortable, form the *Jnana Mudra* by bringing together the tip of your thumb and pointing finger • [Lead through Breath Meditation – see script Week 1]

Uttpluthi   *drishti:* **nose**

Overview	• **Introduce** *Uttpluthi* • **Demonstrate** • **Do it with them and or watch them do it** **NOTE:** • Do this posture with them, watch them do it or do a combination of both • The *drishti* is incorporated in Week 3

Introduce & Demonstrate face-on
 	
Uttpluthi
	• The final working posture demands that we use our *bandhas*
	• This encourages the energy that we have built up in our practice to ascend or move up the central energy channel
	• It is strenuous by very rejuvenating/revitalising
	• It's called *Uttpluthi* or uprooting – you'll see why
	• Move your blanket away
	• Ground your hands
	• Inhale lift your buttocks off the floor
	• Exhale lower down
	    o Try to hold the posture for at least 10 breaths
	        ▪ Let's try that

Do With / Watch Them	• Move your blanket away
	• Ground your hands alongside your hips
	    o Spread your fingers wide
	    o Draw your shoulder blades down away from your ears
	    o Broaden your shoulder blades on your back
	    o Bend your arms slightly so there is space under your armpits and
	• Inhaling lift your buttocks up towards your armpits
	• Hold it there
	• Keep breathing
	• Push the floor away with your hands
	• Keep the head upright
	• Notice that the rate of your breath will increase
	• Exhaling lower your buttocks back down to the mat

Week 3

WEEK 3 • *Drishti & Awareness*

Class Overview	<ul><li>Revise last class and introduce today's class<ul><li>Introduce & teach *drishti*</li><li>Revise *bandhas*</li><li>Lead through 4 *Surya Namaskara A*</li><li>Revise *Surya Namaskara B*<ul><li>3 in total</li></ul></li><li>Talk through *Padangushtasana* & *Pada Hastasana*</li><li>Revise *Trikonasana*</li><li>Teach *Parshvakonasana*<ul><li>Modified version</li></ul></li><li>Teach *Prasarita A, B, C & D*</li><li>Teach a full *Vinyasa* to sitting<ul><li>Basic version</li></ul></li><li>Sitting *asana*</li><li>*Shavasana*</li></ul></li></ul>**NOTE:**<ul><li>Incorporate the *drishti* for each posture</li><li>Include a description of the *bandhas* in each posture as a revision</li></ul>

REVISION: *Bandhas*
<ul><li>Good morning/hello/*Namaste*<ul><li>Any questions on what we have done so far?</li><li>Does everyone understand how to engage the *bandhas* we learnt last week?</li><li>**[For a revision of the *bandhas* see Week 2's script]**</li></ul></li></ul>

Drishti	
Introduction	<ul><li>This week we will learn another important aspect of the yoga practise</li><li>It's something you have already been doing as I've talked you through</li><li>It is where you gaze or position your eyes in each posture<ul><li>This is called *drishti*<ul><li>Some of the gaze positions we have already used are your thumbs when you raise your arms above your head or simply looking upward. Others we'll use are the toes and the tip of your nose.</li></ul></li></ul></li></ul>

	<ul><li>When using the *drishti* it is important to not focus the eyes<ul><li>For example when you gaze toward the tip of your nose, you're not looking at your nose but softly gazing in that direction.<ul><li>Otherwise you may go cross-eyed!</li></ul></li><li>One of my favourite description of *drishti* is from Richard Freeman, he says "It's like nobody looking at nothing in particular"</li></ul></li><li>We use *drishti* because<ul><li>Having a resting place for your eyes diminishes the visual distraction of what's around you</li><li>This encourages our attention inward and</li><li>Helps to develop our awareness of what we're doing, and especially of where we are in space<ul><li>Let's try gazing softly toward the tip of the nose</li></ul></li></ul></li></ul>
Do With / Watch Them	<ul><li>Keep your gaze soft</li><li>Do not focus on your nose but look in that direction<ul><li>You should still have peripheral vision</li><li>Remember, it's like "Nobody looking at nothing in particular"</li></ul></li><li>And relax your gaze</li><li>As we go through the postures today I will continue to point our where the *drishti* is for each posture</li></ul>
Watch Them	<ul><li>Let's start by sitting up tall on your blankets</li><li>Gaze softly down toward the tip of your nose</li><li>Begin to breath fully into the four areas of your chest, the front, the sides, the back and up into the top lobes of your lungs</li><li>Smoothly exhale being sure to make the *ujjayi* sound as you breathe</li><li>Keep breathing fully and</li><li>Gently contract the pelvic floor, creating a lifting sensation at the base of the spine</li><li>Now brace your lower abdomen as if you were about to laugh and feel your lower belly become firm</li><li>Do a couple more rounds of breath</li><li>And relax</li><li>Let's come to standing and apply that to all of our postures</li></ul>
Samasthiti	
Watch Them	<ul><li>Standing in *Samashtiti*<ul><li>**[Choose some instructions from Week 1's script]**</li></ul></li></ul>

Surya Namaskara A	
Introduction & Demonstration	• Maintain *Samasthiti* and watch me as I demonstrate the first sun salutation for you again
Watch Them	• 4x *Surya A* ○ **[Choose some instructions from Week 1's script]**

REVISION: *Surya Namaskara B*	

Overview	• Being a revision only of *Surya Namaskara B* the main differences will be that you can
	  ○ Combine teaching the arms & legs of *Utkatasana*
	  ○ Leave out *Virabhadrasana* from standing
	  ○ Leave out doing the complete *Surya Namaskara B* with them
	• Otherwise, breakdown *Surya Namaskara B* as you did in the last class
	  ○ This is necessary as they make not have done it since last class (weekly students) or you may have a student who missed the second class
	• **Workshop any part not workshopped last week**
	  ○ Or any other aspect that needs refining (eg, squaring the hips in *Virabhadrasana*, etc).
	    • Lead through 3 *Surya Namaskara B*

Introduction	• Did you all get to practice the B version of the sun salutation over the last week? ○ Ok, let's see who really did! • Let's revise some of it
Demonstrate *Utkatasana*	**Arms & legs together** • Inhale, arms up in front, squat low • Exhale, straighten up, hands down through the centre • Remember we entered and exited *Surya Namaskara B* from this posture, the power posture or *Utkatasana*

Do With / Watch Them	• Inhale, drop your sit bones, palms together, arms straight out in front, gaze to your thumbs
	• Exhale, hands down past the heart centre, straighten your legs
	  ○ Again
	• Inhale, deeply bend your knees, shoulders down, raise your arms up in front, gaze up
	• Exhale, lower your hands down the centre, back to *Samashtiti*
	  ○ Once more

	• Inhale, squat low, shoulders heavy, straight arms, palms together, gaze follows your thumbs • Exhale, lower the arms down through the centre, legs straighten

Demonstrate *Virabhadrasana*	**From Downward Dog**
	• The second posture that makes up the sun salutation was the warrior posture or *Virabhadrasana*
	  o Remember we entered this posture from Downward Dog
	  o Watch me again first
	• **[See script Week 2]**

Do With / Watch Them	• **[See script Week 2]**
Demonstrate *Surya Namaskara B*	• **[See script Week 2]**
Watch Them	• [Lead through 3 *Surya Namaskara B*] • **[See script Week 2]**

TALK-THROUGH:	**Standing Postures**
Padangustasana	• **[See Script Week 2]**
Pada Hastasana	• **[See Script Week 2]**
REVISION: *Trikonasana*	

Trikonasana	• Do you remember the new standing posture we learnt last week?
	• Let me show you again
	  o **[Demonstrate]**
	• Let me see you do it
	  o **[Watch them]**
	• **[See script Week 2]**

Parshvakonasana Modification   *drishti:* ceiling / inside of elbow

Overview	- Introduce *Parshvakonasana* - Demonstrate - Teach hip action - Workshop knee position - Teach arm action - Teach complete posture **NOTE:** - Teach the legs and arm actions separately - Having students turn their palms to face upward makes it easier for them to get their shoulder into the correct position - The 'Shoulder Option' should only be given on an individual basis for those who are too stiff to take their arm up into position - The *drishti* is modified to the ceiling or elbow
Intro	- The new posture we'll learn this week is called *Parshvakonasana*, which simply means the side-angle posture, you'll soon see why.

Demonstrate face-on	- *Samasthiti*
	- Inhale, hands to *Namaste*, wide stance
	- Exhale, arms shoulder height
	- Inhale right foot 90 degrees, left toes in slightly
	- Exhale, bend the knee
	- Inhale, roll the palms to face up
	- Exhale, elbow to knee, arm overhead
	  - 5 breaths here
	- Inhale, come up
	- Exhale, straighten the feet
	  - The other side
	- Inhale, left foot 90 degrees, right foot in slightly
	- Exhale, knee above the ankle
	- Inhale, turn the palms up
	- Exhale, elbow to knee, arm overhead
	  - Gaze to the ceiling for 5 breaths
	- Inhale, straighten the leg to come up
	- Exhale, back to *Samashtiti*
	  - Let's break that up a little

Workshop Hips	- Let's look at what we do with our hips and legs
	- The stance for this posture will be your widest for all of the standing postures
	  - Like the warrior posture, it needs be wide enough that you can work deeply into it without your knee moving beyond your ankle
	    - Work toward having your thigh parallel to the floor
	  - So again, to protect your knee check that it hovers above your ankle joint and does not sit above your toes
	- Be precise with your feet and line them up to do the right side first
	  - Right foot 90 degrees, left toes turn in slightly

	- Now, when you bend the right knee, drop your weight in the centre so that you do not unearth the outside of the left foot *
	    o The little-toe-side of your left foot must still touch the mat
	    o This means continuing to work the left leg as strongly as the right
	    o You should feel a sense of buoyancy under your hips
	- With the knee bent, work the groins open/ knees away from each other
	- Check that your knee tracks over the ankle and does not fall forward of the knee
	
	* To check that too much weight is not being borne into the foot of the bent leg, get students to check if they can lift the front of that foot off the floor. If all the weight is borne onto that foot they will not be able to lift the front of the foot off the floor

Workshop Arms	- Now let's look at the arm position
	- **[Demonstrate with leg position]**
	- We turn our palms up to face the ceiling
	- And we simply raise our left arm up above our head
	- The right arm bends so our elbow rests on our knee
	    o Let your top arm continue the line of your leg and torso
	    o If it's comfortable, gaze up to the ceiling/the inside of your elbow
	- Inhale come up and try the other side
	    o Your turn

Do With / Watch Them	- Standing in *Samasthiti*
	- Inhale, hands to your chest in *Namaste*
	- Exhale take a wide step to your right
	    o Adjust your stance here if you need to
	- Arms out at shoulder height
	- Keep breathing and your arms out at shoulder height
	    o Now position your right foot at 90 degrees and turn your left foot in slightly
	    o Keep your torso upright in the centre so that your weight is equally distributed into both feet
	    o Now bend your right knee as deeply as you can, adjusting your stance again if necessary, so your knee does not extend beyond your ankle
	    o Keep your left leg strong and straight and work your right knee back to open your groins
	- Inhale roll your arms to have your palms face up to the ceiling
	- Exhale lower the right arm to rest your elbow on your knee
	- Inhale look up to the ceiling and raise your left arm up over your head
	    o Holding this position, we'll work the posture for 5 breaths
	    o Check you still have weight in the left foot with the little toe side of your foot grounded/making contact with the mat
	    o Both *bandhas* engaged, lifting the pelvic floor and the lower abdomen engaged/braced/firm
	    o Keep your shoulders down away from your ears, the left armpit works towards the floor, palm faces the floor

	<ul><li>○ Lift your heart, shoulders down, back of the neck long</li></ul><ul><li>Inhaling, push off your right foot and come upright</li><li>Exhale, arms out shoulder height, gaze straight ahead</li><li>Inhale, change your feet, right 90 degrees, left in slightly</li><li>Exhale keep weight in both feet, bend the left knee</li><li>Inhale work your left knee back to open your groins</li><li>Exhale, roll your palms to face the ceiling</li><li>Inhale lift out of your hips, lift your heart</li><li>Exhale lower the left elbow to your left thigh</li><li>Inhale reach the right arm up over your head, gaze to the ceiling<ul><li>○ Continue to push off the left foot to transfer weight back into the right foot</li><li>○ Do not collapse into the left hip but keep your hips buoyant away from the floor</li><li>○ Keep a lifting sensation from your insteps, up into your torso and along the entire length of your spine and neck</li><li>○ Work the right hand away from the right foot and your right foot away from your right hand</li><li>○ Keep breath full and directed, moving your chest in all directions</li></ul></li><li>Inhaling, push off the left foot to bring yourself upright</li><li>Exhale square off your feet and step or hop back to *Samasthiti*</li></ul>
Shoulder Option	**[For those students whose shoulders are too stiff to take into position]**<ul><li>Keeping the arm straight take your arm down toward the floor and raise it up past your face to come up over your head</li></ul>

Prasarita Padottanasana A, B, C & D	drishti: nose
Overview	<ul><li>**Introduce the *Prasaritas***</li><li>**Demonstrate A & B**</li><li>**Watch them do it**<ul><li>○ **Workshop stance & feet**</li></ul></li><li>**Demonstrate C & D**<ul><li>○ **Workshop the arms for C**</li></ul></li><li>**Watch them do it**</li></ul>**NOTE**:<ul><li>Students with low blood pressure may experience dizziness in this posture. Give them the alternative of taking an additional breath on the way up.</li><li>Be careful to not demonstrate these postures with your back to students, you may need to angle your position.</li><li>You do not need to do bend forward into the posture with students. Once forward they will not be able to see you. Instead, watch them.</li><li>In *Prasarita A & D* the arms are not extended out to the side before going forward. Instead, after going forward and before coming up, an extra inhalation is inserted.</li><li></li></ul>

	- In *Prasarita B & C* the arms are extended out to the side before going forward. We then go straight forward into the posture and straight up out of the posture. - Teach A & B, then C & D separately as many beginners will find it difficult to hold a wide-legged stance for the duration of both
Introduction	- The next standing posture we'll learn has four variations - I'll demonstrate A and B first and then get you to do them - Then we'll learn C and D o Watch me
Demonstrate side-on	**[Demonstrate with bent knees]** - From *Samasthiti* - Inhale, step to the right, medium stance - Exhale, hands to your hips - Inhale, look up - Exhale, fold forward, hand to the floor - Inhale, lift and look up - Exhale, forward for 5 breaths - Inhale, look up - Exhale, hands to the hips - Inhale, come up **B version** - Inhale, arms extend out - Exhale, hands to your hips - Inhale, look up - Exhale, fold forward for 5 breaths - Inhale, come all the way up - Exhale, back to *Samasthiti* o Ok, let me see you do that

Watch Them	**A version**
	- From *Samasthiti*
	- Inhale, step to the right
	- Exhale, hands to your hips
	  o Look down to your feet and adjust them so the outside edges of your feet are parallel
	  o The distance of your feet is shorter than for the last posture
	  o It is important that your stance is not too short
	    ▪ Or it will be a long way to the floor!
	  o Or too wide
	    ▪ As this makes it difficult to hold
	  o Adjust your stance if you need to
	- Ground the four corners of your feet, lift your insteps, your kneecaps and the pelvic floor
	- With your low abdomen firm
	- Inhale, lift your heart and look up
	- Exhale fold forward bending your knees as your need to, hands to the floor
	- Inhale lift your chest, broaden your shoulders

	- Exhale fold forward, hands to the floor between your feet
    - 5 full, directed breaths here, notice your ribs move as you breathe
    - Check that your hands are straight and shoulder-width apart, spread your fingers wide
    - Lift your shoulders away from the floor and draw your shoulder blades up to your hips
    - Lengthen your spine and neck, keep them relaxed
    - Gaze toward the tip of your nose, keep the gaze soft
- Inhale lift your chest and head and look up
- Stay there and exhaling place your hands on your hips
- Inhale, strong legs and come on up
- Exhale stay there

B version
- Inhale, keep the action in your feet and legs and extend your arms out shoulder height
- Exhale, hands to your hips
- Inhale, lift up out of your feet
- Exhale, fold forward
    - Gaze softly toward the tip of the nose
    - Keep your feet active and your legs strong
    - Lift pelvic floor and with your fingers feel the lower belly firm
    - Release your spine and neck toward the floor
    - Actively lift your shoulders away from your ears
- Inhale leading with your head, lift your torso and come upright
    - If this makes you light-headed take an extra breath to come up
- Exhale, come back to *Samasthiti* |
| **Demonstrate & Workshop** | - Now I'll show you the C and D versions
[Demonstrate arms only back-on, turn to side or face-on to bend forward]
- Inhale, arms out shoulder height
- Exhale, hands behind your back
    - Interlace your fingers
    - It is important here to roll the shoulders back and
    - Attempt to straighten the elbows/arms
    - Maintain this position with your arms
- Inhale, look up
- Exhale, fold forward for 5 breaths
- Inhale, come all the way up
- Exhale, hands to hips

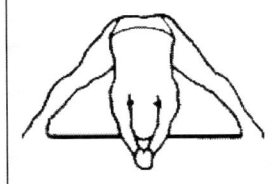

D version
- Inhale, look up
- Exhale, fold forward, pick up the big toes
- Inhale, lift and look up
- Exhale, forward for 5 breaths
- Inhale, look up
- Exhale, hands to the hips
- Inhale, come up
- Exhale, *Samasthiti*
    - Your turn |

Do With / Watch Them	**C version**
	• From *Samasthiti*
	• Inhale, step to the right
	• Exhale, hands to your hips
	    o Again check that the outside edges of your feet are parallel and
	    o Your feet are the right distance apart for you
	• Inhaling, extend your arms out to shoulder height
	• Exhaling, hands behind your back
	• **[Do arms with them, back-on]**
	    o Now interlace your fingers
	    o Roll your shoulders firmly back and
	    o Work towards straightening out your elbows/arms
	    o Keep your arms here, breathe in and
	• Exhale, fold forward
	    o *Drishti* again is toward the tip of the nose
	    o Keep working the arms straight and release your shoulders
	    o Remember to bend your knees if you feel your low back round
	    o Try to recreate the curve in your low back
	    o Splay your sit bones wide and up to the ceiling
	• Inhale, lift your head first and slowly come to upright
	
	D version
	• Inhaling, lift from the insteps of your feet
	• Exhaling, strong legs, fold forward
	• Now pick up your big toes with your first two fingers and thumb
	• Inhaling lift your heart, broad shoulders
	• Exhale fold forward
	    o Return your gaze toward the tip of your nose
	    o Neck in line with the rest of your spine
	    o Lift your shoulders and elbows toward the ceiling
	    o Keep the low belly firm, the pelvic floor lifted
	    o Sit bones wide and working toward the ceiling, strong legs
	• Inhale lift your heart and gaze upward
	• Stay forward, exhale hands to your hips
	• Inhale, slowly come up
	• Exhale, step back to *Samashtiti*

Vinyasa - Basic

Overview	• **Introduce *Vinyasa***
	• **Demonstrate a full *Vinyasa***
	• **Do it with them**
	    o From standing or Downward Dog
	• **Watch them**
	    o Repeat a few times from Downward Dog in their own time
	• **Workshop as necessary**

	NOTE:
	- If this is not possible give the alternative 'easy' version to sitting. Only give this version to those who need it.
	- Allow students to try a few in their own time
	- Give alternative (Easy) version only to those who need it

Introduction	- In Ashtanga Yoga all the postures are connected by sequential movements that are synchronised with the breath
	   o This is called a *vinyasa*
	
	- So in order to go from our standing postures to our sitting postures we use a sequence of movements, each movement synchronised with a phase of our breath
	- The good news is that you already know most of these movements
	   o They are the basis of our sun salutations
	      ▪ I'll show you how we use them to transit from standing to sitting…

Demonstrate side-on	- Inhale, arms up
	- Exhale, forward
	- Inhale, lift
	- Exhale, Rod
	- Inhale, Upward Dog
	- Exhale, Downward Dog
	   o From here bring one leg up [between your hands]
	      ▪ Foot pointed
	      ▪ Knee to the mat
	   o Bring the other leg up behind
	      ▪ Cross the ankles
	      ▪ Knees close together
	   o Flex the feet, push off your hands and sit down
	   o Stretch the legs out to sitting
	      ▪ Let's try that

Do With / Watch Them	- Inhale, arms up, gaze up
	- Exhale, forward from your hips
	- Inhale, lift your heart
	- Exhale, step back to Rod
	- Inhale, pull your heart through to Upward Dog
	- Exhale, Downward Dog
	   o At the end of your exhalation, bend your knees, look to your thumbs
	- Keep breathing
	- Point one foot and bring your knee to the floor between your hands
	- Point the other foot and draw the knee up behind the first
	- Knees close together on the mat
	- Now flex the feet, toes point out to the side
	- Gently push off your hands, back onto your buttocks
	- Stretch your legs out in front
	   o Play with that a couple of times from Downward Dog in your own time

Workshop	<ul><li>**Feet**<ul><li>Everyone try with me to point your foot and now flex your foot</li><li>**[Demonstrate & do it with them]**</li><li>Now please listen carefully for the right queue<ul><li>It is really important to point your feet as you bring them forward, otherwise you won't be able to get your knees to the floor</li><li>And it is equally important to flex the feet when I instruct you, otherwise you will find it hard to sit back down</li></ul></li></ul></li><li>**Knees**<ul><li>With your ankles crossed keep your knees close together and</li><li>Step far enough up that your knees come between your hands</li></ul></li><li>**Alternative (Easy version)**<ul><li>Bring one knee up between the hands</li><li>Bring the second knee to meet it, so you are kneeling</li><li>Sit back onto your heels</li><li>Gently swing your legs around to the front</li></ul></li></ul>

Week 4

WEEK 4 • The 8 Limbs

Class Overview	• Greeting, revision last class, introduction of today's class
	   o **Explain the 8 Limbs of Yoga**
	      ▪ Lead through *3 Surya Namaskara A*
	   o **Teach lowering down in the Rod**
	      ▪ Lead through *2 more Surya Namaskara A*
	      ▪ Lead through *3 Surya Namaskara B x 3*
	   o **Lead through *Padangushtasana, Pada Hastasana & Trikonasana***
	   o Revise *Parshvakonasana*
	   o Revise *Prasarita A, B, C & D*
	   o **Teach *Parshvottanasana***
	   o **Teach *UHP* Preparation**
	   o **Teach the Warrior sequence**
	   o **Teach *Vinyasa* to sitting (Stepping)**
	   o **Finishing sitting postures & *Shavasana***
	
	NOTE:
	• Before teaching lowering down in the Rod, warm them up with 3 *Surya Namaskara A*
	• Incorporate the *drishti* for each posture
	• Include a description of the *bandhas* in each posture

8 Limbs of Yoga	

Overview	**NOTE:**
	• Below is a possible script which can also be used as a guide
	   o Make your description of the limbs relatable
	   o Keep it simple - this is not a philosophy lecture!
	   o With the *yamas* and *niyamas*, you can either list them all, or just give one as an example and elaborate on it
	   o Do not say anything you do not understand yourself – it will show
	• Always refer the students to Gregor's book should they would wish to explore the eight limbs further.
	• Gregor Maehle's 'Ashtanga Yoga, Practice & Philosophy' book is a great resource should you wish to write your own script

Introduction	• Good morning/hello/*Namaste* everyone
	   o How did you go practising during the week?
	   o Any questions on anything so far?
	
	• I'd like to take five minutes today to give you an overview of the eight limbs of yoga
	   o *Ashtanga* means eight limbs - nothing to do with arms and legs!

- This eight-limbed system was devised thousands of years ago by an Indian sage, named *Patanjali*. The eight limbs was his system to help human beings move from suffering to freedom, from pain to joy and from ignorance to realisation
    - I'll give you a brief description of what these eight limbs are

- The first limb is called **yama** or restraints. There are five *yama*s and they address the way a person relates to other people and the world around them. In the western world, *yama*s are very similar to what we call 'common law'.
    - One example of a *yama* is non-violence. Most of you will have noticed that violence rarely, if ever, leads to a positive outcome of a situation. The *yama* of non-violence suggests that if anger arises within a person, they are best to restrain themselves from becoming violent. The *yama*s are designed to create a basic level of peace within society.

    OR
    - The five *yama*s are: non-violence, truthfulness, non-stealing, sexual restraint and non-greed. My favourite of these in non-greed. Non-greed is not consuming more than we need. Our society encourages us to be greedy, to indulge ourselves, pamper ourselves, shop 'til you drop, etc. After all "you deserve it", don't you? Greed is the opposite of contentment.

- The second limb is **niyama**. The *niyama*s refer to observances that relate to a persons inner world or their relationship with themselves. Just as the *yama*s create peace within the wider society, the *niyama*s create a basic level of peace within the individual.
    - There are also five *niyama*s. These are cleanliness, contentment, simplicity, self-study and the recognition of a Supreme Being or a power greater than ourselves.
    - Contentment in yogic scriptures is described as 'the greatest happiness'. Contentment is being satisfied and happy with what we have, however great or small. This enables one to be happy regardless of wealth or status. In our competitive society contentment may have become a foreign concept.

- The third limb is **asana**. *Asana* means posture or the practice of physical yoga exercises. This is the limb that yoga is known for in the west. Through the practice of *asana*, the body becomes healthy, strong and flexible. This enables a person to perform their daily duties with ease and eventually to sit in mediation without discomfort or physical fatigue.

- The fourth limb of yoga is **pranayama**. An example of a *pranayama* technique is the *Ujjayi pranayama* that you learnt in the first week of the course. Ancient Indian yogis noticed that the breath had a significant effect on the body and the mind. Through the usage of certain breathing techniques they realised that it is possible to tame the mind and balance the nervous system. *Pranayama* purifies and calms the mind.

- The fifth limb is called *pratyahara*. This means the withdrawal of the senses from external phenomena so that one can be guided by their inner knowing rather than being continually distracted by external events and circumstances. Examples of *pratyahara* techniques are the *drishti* or gaze point and listening to the sound of your breath in the *Ujjayi pranayama* as we withdraw the senses of sight and sound, respectively. *Pratyahara* techniques inspire one to lead a more internally motivated life.

- The sixth limb is **dharana** or concentration. This is the ability to focus the mind on an object, such as the breath, without being distracted. After a certain amount of time concentrating on an object, the mind becomes completely silent and then enters into the seventh limb…

- Which is **dhyana**, more commonly known as meditation. The difference between concentration and meditation is that the subject, (the person meditating) and the object (for example, the breath) have become one. There is no experience of separation between the observer and that being observed.

- The eighth limb is called **samadhi**. This limb is not something that is practiced, as such, but arises naturally when a person has practiced the preceding limbs and is able to remain in meditation for long periods of time. *Samadhi* is the ultimate flowering of human potential and just as a flower cannot be forced to open early, a human being cannot force *samadhi* to happen but can only enter a meditative state and allow it to unfold naturally. Some common experiences associated with the state of *samadhi* are: feelings of bliss and infinite peace, an ending of all fear and suffering, total inability to be distracted, increased creativity, effortless health and ease of living.

- Hopefully that has given you some insight into the eight-limbed Ashtanga Yoga system

- If you would like to explore the eight limbs further, Gregor's book 'Ashtanga Yoga, Practice & Philosophy' is an excellent resource

Lowering Down in Sun Salutations

Overview	<ul><li>Introduce lowering down into the Rod as an option</li><li>Demonstrate lowering down into Rod posture<ul><li>Demonstrate elbows in close to waist</li><li>Demonstrate on knees</li></ul></li><li>Get all to do on knees<ul><li>Explain this is 'the Rod'</li></ul></li><li>Give option to include in sun salutations sometimes or always</li></ul>

	NOTE: • Be sure students are warmed up with at least 3 *Surya Namaskara A* before teaching them to lower down into the Rod.
Introduction	• OK, so who of you find the Rod easy? • Good, we have a variation which you can do if you would like a further challenge o I'll show you how

Demonstrate	**[Side-on]**
	• In Rod
	• Exhale, lower down
	
	[Face-on]
	• It's really important to keep your elbows tucked in to/hugging the waist
	• From the front you'll see my elbows stay in close to my sides
	
	[On knees]
	• So you can focus on the correct shoulder action, let's try it on our knees - that way there's less weight in your hands and you can test out your strength
	   o From Rod
	   o Bend the knees
	   o Elbows in close
	   o Exhale, lower down
	• Let's try that together

**Do With /
Watch Them**
	• Let's start on our knees with your shoulders above your wrists
	• Keep your *ujjayi* breath going
	   o Now check that you hands are shoulder-width apart
	      ▪ Fingers spread wide
	      ▪ Middle finger points straight ahead
	      ▪ Keep the base of each finger and the heel of your hand grounded
	   o Draw your shoulder blades down your back and
	   o Draw the sternum forward
	   o Step your feet back into a long, strong Rod
	   o Now bend both knees down onto the mat
	      ▪ Inhale, keep the elbows hugging your sides
	      ▪ Exhale, lower your chest between your arms
	         - Don't jut the chin forward/ Keep your ears back in line with your shoulders
	      ▪ Inhale straighten your arms
	      ▪ Exhale and relax
	• If you found that too difficult, stay with keeping your arms straight or bend the arms a little
	• If you found that easy enough, you can try the same thing with your legs straight
	   o So you'll lower down from a Rod
	• Let's do that once more

	<ul><li>○ Either do the original version of Rod, keeping the arms straight or</li><li>○ Lower down from a straight-legged Rod<ul><li>■ It is important to not compromise the correct action with your shoulders otherwise you will never develop the strength you need</li></ul></li></ul><ul><li>In the following sun salutations, when I call the Rod, you can choose either of these options or you can vary them</li><li>Please listen to your body and go at your own pace</li></ul>

REVISION: *Parshvakonasana* Modification

Overview	<ul><li>Demonstrate and revise complete posture without the hip and arm breakdown</li><li>See Script Week 3</li></ul>

REVISION: *Prasarita Padottanasana* A, B, C & D

Overview	<ul><li>Introduce the *Prasaritas*</li><li>Demonstrate ABC & D together</li><li>You do not need to do the variations with them as they are relatively simple</li><li>Watch them do the postures</li></ul>
Introduction	<ul><li>Last week the new standing posture we learnt had an A, B, C and D version<ul><li>○ Do you remember it?</li></ul></li><li>This week we'll put the four together<ul><li>○ Watch me first</li></ul></li><li>[See script from Week 3]</li></ul>

Parshvottanasana   *drishti:* nose

Overview	<ul><li>Introduce *Parshvottanasana*</li><li>Demonstrate arms only<ul><li>○ Both arms at the same time</li><li>○ One arm at a time</li><li>○ Alternative - hold the elbows</li></ul></li><li>Demonstrate feet & squaring hips only</li><li>Demonstrate arm & hips combined with folding forward<ul><li>○ For each: do with them & watch them do it</li></ul></li></ul>

Introduction	• In the next standing posture we're going to do a forward bend with our hands on our back in a prayer position!
	    ○ We'll learn the arms first and then the hip position
	        ▪ Watch me

Demonstrate back-on ARMS	**Arms**
	• **There are a few options to get your arms into position**
	• We can take both arms together into position
	    ○ Arms out shoulder height
	    ○ Roll the arms forward
	    ○ Hands behind the back
	    ○ And bring them together into prayer on your back
	    ○ To come out, release the arms and extend them out at shoulder height
	• The other option is to take one hand at a time into position
	    ○ Arms are out at shoulder height
	    ○ Again, roll the arms forward
	    ○ Bend the right elbow
	    ○ Take the hand behind the back
	    ○ Take the second hand into position
	    ○ Palms together on your back
	    ○ Come out and extend the arms out at shoulder height
	• If you can't get your arms into position with those options
	    ○ Simply take your hands behind your back and
	    ○ Grasp the elbows
	        ▪ Let's try that together

Do With / Watch Them	• **[Optional: start from *Samasthiti*]** • Extend your arms out shoulder height • Now roll your arms forward so your palms face backward • Either one arm at a time or both arms together, take your hands into prayer position on your back ○ If you can't make that, hold your elbows behind your back • Now roll your shoulder back and • Draw the elbows toward each other / Lift the elbows off your back

Demonstrate side-on FEET & HIPS	**Feet & Hips**
	• Now I'll show you what we do with the feet and hips…
	• This posture will have the shortest stance of all the standing postures
	    ○ Inhale, step to the right, landing in a short stance
	    ○ Exhale, hands to the hips
	    ○ Inhale, right foot opens 90 degrees and
	    ○ Exhaling, squaring to the right foot, left foot at 45 degrees
	    ○ Inhale lift out of the hips
	    ○ Exhale fold forward along the front leg
	        ▪ 5 breaths here
	        ▪ Fractionally bend the knee
	    ○ Inhaling, head first, come up
	    ○ Turn your feet to the left side
	    ○ Square off

	<ul><li>○ Inhale look up</li><li>○ Exhale forward<ul><li>▪ 5 breaths</li><li>▪ Drop the chin</li></ul></li><li>○ Inhale head first to come up</li><li>○ Exhale *Samasthiti*<ul><li>▪ Let's try that</li></ul></li></ul>
Do With / Watch Them	<ul><li>Inhale hands to *Namaste*</li><li>Exhale step your feet to the right, landing in a short stance (the shortest stance so far), hands to your hips<ul><li>○ Open your right foot to 90 degrees</li><li>○ Swivel on your back foot, to square your hips and shoulders to the right foot/short edge of your mat</li></ul></li><li>Your back/left foot should be at a 45 degree angle<ul><li>○ Look back to check and adjust your foot as necessary</li></ul></li><li>Now look at your hands and try to bring them to the same level<ul><li>○ Work the left hip forward, the right hip back to square the hips</li><li>○ Lightly squeeze the thighs together to keep your balance</li></ul></li><li>Inhale lift out of your hips</li><li>Exhale fold forward over the right leg<ul><li>○ Drop you chin so your head is in line with the rest of your spine</li><li>○ Fractionally bend the front knee</li></ul></li><li>Inhale, lead with your head to come up</li><li>To change sides turn your feet and torso to the opposite side</li><li>Now open your left foot at 90 degrees and your right foot at 45 degrees as you square off to the left foot<ul><li>○ Spike down the back heel and</li><li>○ Ground the inside of the front foot</li></ul></li><li>Inhale strong legs</li><li>Exhale fold forward over the front leg<ul><li>○ Drop the chin to remove any creases from the back of your neck</li><li>○ Keep the legs working strongly</li><li>○ Fractionally bend the front knee</li></ul></li><li>Inhale, head first, come up</li><li>Square off to the long edge of the mat</li><li>Exhale back to *Samasthiti*</li></ul>
Demonstrate side-on FULL POSTURE	**[Start demonstration back-on to show arm action]**<ul><li>OK, watch me as I do the complete posture<ul><li>○ Inhale, step to the right, short stance</li><li>○ Exhale, arms shoulder height</li><li>○ Roll the arms forward and hands into prayer or hold the elbows</li><li>○ Inhale, right foot 90 degrees</li><li>○ Exhale, square off, left foot 45 degrees</li><li>○ Inhale, lift, look up</li><li>○ Exhale forward<ul><li>▪ 5 breaths</li><li>▪ Gaze to the toes</li><li>▪ Elbows lift</li><li>▪ Bend the knee</li></ul></li><li>○ Inhale, head first, come up</li><li>○</li></ul></li></ul>

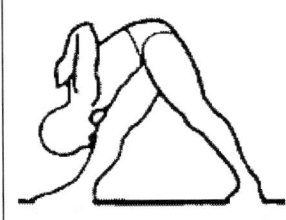

	<ul><li>Exhale turn your feet, hips and shoulders to the left</li><li>Inhale, left foot 90</li><li>Exhale, square off, right foot 45 degrees</li><li>Inhale, lift</li><li>Exhale forward<ul><li>5 breaths here</li><li>Drop the chin</li><li>Bend the knee</li></ul></li><li>Inhale, come up, release the arms</li><li>Exhale, *Samashtiti*<ul><li>Any questions?</li><li>Are you ready to try that together?</li></ul></li></ul>
Do With / Watch Them	<ul><li>*Samasthiti*, inhale hands up to *Namaste*, step your feet to the right</li><li>Exhale, landing in the shortest stance for all of our standing postures</li><li>Extend your arms out shoulder height and roll your arms forward so your palms face backward<ul><li>Now, either one arm at a time or both arms together, take your hands into prayer on your back, otherwise clasp your elbows</li><li>Roll your shoulder back and lift the elbows toward each other</li></ul></li><li>Keeping your arms in position<ul><li>Turn your right foot open to 90 degrees</li><li>Swivel on your back foot to square your hips and shoulders to the right foot/short edge of your mat</li><li>Your back/left foot grounds down at a 45 degree angle</li></ul></li><li>Inhale, lightly squeeze the thighs together, lift up out of your hips</li><li>Exhale keep the heart lifted as you fold forward<ul><li>5 breaths gazing toward your toes</li><li>Keep the base of your right big toe grounding, the heel of the back foot spikes down</li><li>Both legs are strong and straight. Do not lock out the front knee</li><li>Lift your elbows away from the floor</li><li>Keep the spine and neck long, drop your chin</li></ul></li><li>Inhale, fractionally bend the front knee, lead with your head, come up</li><li>Exhale turn your feet, hips and shoulders to the left side</li><li>Take a breath here to check that your hips are square and your back foot is at a 45 degree angle</li><li>Inhale feet grounding, lift your heart</li><li>Exhale, strong legs and fold forward<ul><li>If you are unsteady, lightly squeeze the thighs together</li><li>Keep the back heel and base of the front big toe firmly grounded</li><li>Lift your elbows away from the floor, the heart stays lifted</li><li>With the pelvic floor and lower abdomen engaged, lengthen your entire spine</li><li>Take any creases out of the back of your neck and gaze to your toes</li></ul></li><li>Inhale, keep the heart lifted as you come up</li><li>Exhale square off your feet, extend your arms out and step back to *Samasthiti*</li></ul>

Utthita Hasta Padangushtasana (UHP) **Preparation**

Overview	- **Introduce balancing**
	- **Demonstrate**
	- **Do it with them – right side**
	- **Watch them do it – left side**
	
	NOTE:
	- This is a preparation posture for UHP - the knee is kept bent until the final position
	  - The objective is to teach students to balance without the added challenge of needing adequate flexibility to do the final posture
	- Keep the breaths shorter as these are strenuous positions
	- There is no need to repeat this posture
	  - Do it with them on the right side
	  - Watch them do it for the left side

Introduction	- Our next new posture is a balancing posture, where we stand on one leg
	- The balancing postures teach us how to focus our attention/awareness
	  - Everyone can stand on one foot for at least one second
	  - To maintain that for 5 breaths and then change the position of our leg and/or gaze requires that you keep doing what you did to balance for one second
	  - This requires honing your attention skills
	- Here's a tip: when you attempt to stand on one leg, notice that you'll always fall to the outside of your foot
	- So grounding the inside of the foot will help to prevent that
	  - I'll show you what we're going to do

Demonstrate face-on	- Standing in *Samashtiti*
	- Shift all your weight into the left leg
	- Inhale, lift the right knee to the chest with both hands
	- Exhale, left hand to the hip
	  - 5 breaths here
	- Inhale, lift the knee a little higher
	- Exhale, take the knee out to the right
	  - Gaze shifts to the left
	  - 5 breaths
	- Inhale, knee and gaze back to centre
	- Exhale, extend the leg
	  - 5 breaths here
	- Exhale, lower the leg
	- And repeat on the left side
	  - Let's do that together

Do With / Watch Them	- Standing in *Samashtiti*
- Shift your weight into your left foot and
- Inhale lift your right foot and draw the knee to your chest with both hands
- Exhale place your left hand to your left hip
  - Lengthen through the inseam/inside of your standing leg grounding the inside corners of your foot
  - Keep your gaze steady to the floor or out in front of you
  - Keep your *bandhas* engaged, your low belly firm
  - Drop your shoulders and lengthen your neck
  - Keep breathing
- Inhale lift your knee a little higher and
- Exhale stay focused on your grounded foot as you take the knee to the right
  - Only if you feel steady, turn your head and gaze to the left
  - Check that your torso remains upright
  - Lift out of your hips, heart lifted, chest open
  - Try to keep your breath full and directed
  - Stay focused and now
- Inhaling bring the knee and gaze back to centre
- Exhale both hands to your hips
- Inhaling keep your knee lifting as high as you can and
- Exhale straighten your leg
  - Inside of the right foot grounding
  - Low belly braced
  - Heart lifted
  - Shoulders down
  - Soft gaze
- Exhaling lower your right leg

- **[For the left side use or modify any of the above descriptions or other appropriate instructions]** |

Warrior Sequence

Overview	- **Introduce the Warrior Sequence**
- **Demonstrate the full sequence to Downward Dog**
- **Re-demonstrate transit from *Virabhadrasana* A to B**
  - **Do not hold each posture for 5 breaths but step it through only**
- **Do the transitions with them, watch them do the rest**

NOTE:
- Demonstrate to Downward Dog only. Give students a rest while you teach stepping through to sitting
- Caution! When demonstrating be sure you will still be facing them (versus your back to them) when you transit from *Virabhadrasana A* to *Virabhadrasana B*
- Include both options of lowering down and not lowering down in your demonstrations of the Rod |

	• As most of this is familiar you do not need to do all of it with them. Instead, watch them do the vinyasa parts and do the warrior postures with them. Check that you are facing them, that they can see you, and you can watch them at the same time • The Warrior sequence is very strenuous – be careful to not hold students in the warrior postures for too long. For this same reason, students should only do the complete sequence once through.

Introduction	• The next postures we're going to learn look like a short sequence. Actually it is a *Vinyasa* to *Utkatasana*, our power posture from the B sun salutation, and then another *Vinyasa* to the warrior posture, also from *Surya Namaskara B*.
	   ○ Because this short sequence contains two different warrior postures it is often referred to as the 'Warrior Sequence'
	      ▪ Let me demonstrate it for you
	OR
	• Now we're going to learn a sequence that looks like a *Suryanamaskara A* that flows into *Suryanamaskara* B with an extra warrior posture
	   ○ Because this short sequence contains two different warrior postures it is often referred to as the 'Warrior Sequence'
	      ▪ I'll demonstrate it for you to show you what I mean

Demonstrate FULL SEQUENCE	• *Samashtiti*
	• Full *Vinyasa* OR Like *Surya Namaskara A*
	  ○ Inhale, arms up, gaze up
	  ○ Exhale, fold forward
	  ○ Inhale, lift the heart
	  ○ Exhale, step back to Rod
	  ○ Inhale, Upward Dog
	  ○ Exhale, Downward Dog
	  ○ Inhale, step up and lift
	  ○ Exhale, drop the sit bones into *Utkatasana*
	     ▪ 5 breaths here
	• Full *Vinyasa* OR Like *Surya Namaskara B*
	  ○ Exhale, fold forward
	  ○ Inhale, lift, gaze up
	     ▪ Exhale, Rod
	     ▪ Inhale, Upward Dog
	     ▪ Exhale, Downward Dog
	     ▪ Inhale, right foot up
	     ▪ Exhale, square hips
	     ▪ Inhale, arms up into warrior posture
	        - 5 breaths here
	     ▪ Now watch - we change sides
	  ○ Gaze straight ahead
	  ○ Inhale, up and over to the left
	  ○ Exhale, repeat *Virabhadrasana A*
	     ▪ 5 breaths here
	  ○ Again, watch - transit to *Virabhadrasana B*
	  ○ Exhale hands above the feet
	  ○ Open the hips and chest

	<ul><li>○ Adjust the feet, stance widens<ul><li>▪ 5 breaths here</li></ul></li><li>○ Inhale come up and change sides</li><li>○ Exhale, repeat on the other side<ul><li>▪ 5 breaths</li></ul></li><li>○ Exhale, hands down, step back to Rod</li><li>○ Inhale, Upward Dog</li><li>○ Exhale, Downward Dog</li><li>○ Bend your knees, come to sitting</li></ul>
Re-Demonstrate TRANSIT *Virabhadrasana A → B*	<ul><li>So the only part of this that is new is the B version of the warrior posture</li><li>The only part that is tricky is the transit from *Virabhadrasana A to B*<ul><li>○ I'll re-demonstrate that part and then we'll do that part together</li></ul></li></ul>**[Do not hold warrior postures for 5 breaths, step through only]**<ul><li>○ After 5 breaths in *Virabhadrasana A*<ul><li>▪ Inhale come up and change sides</li></ul></li><li>○ Exhale, over to the left and repeat Warrior A<ul><li>▪ Keep your arms up if you can, otherwise lower them shoulder height</li></ul></li><li>○ Then transit to *Virabhadrasana* or Warrior B</li><li>○ Exhale lower your arms, hands above the feet</li><li>○ Open the hips and chest</li><li>○ Lengthen your stance, adjust your feet</li><li>○ And again up and over to the other side<ul><li>▪ Let's try that together</li></ul></li></ul>
Do With / Watch Them	<ul><li>From *Virabhadrasana A* we change sides<ul><li>○ Gaze straight ahead</li><li>○ Inhale come up, straighten off the feet</li><li>○ Exhale, adjust your feet to the left and repeat Warrior A</li><li>○ Now transit to *Virabhadrasana B*</li><li>○ Exhale lower the arms</li><li>○ Hands hover above the feet</li><li>○ Open the hips and chest to the long edge of your mat</li><li>○ Adjust your feet, widen your stance,</li><li>○ Gaze to the left hand</li><li>○ Inhale up and over to the other side</li><li>○ Adjust your feet</li><li>○ Switch your gaze to the other hand</li><li>○ Exhale and release the posture<ul><li>▪ Let's try that bit, then we'll do the whole sequence</li></ul></li></ul></li></ul>
FULL SEQUENCE **Do With / Watch Them**	<ul><li>Standing in *Samasthiti*<ul><li>○ Ground your feet, strong legs, lift from the pelvic floor, brace your lower abdomen, open the front and back of your heart area, shoulders down, back of the neck long</li><li>○ Establish you *ujjayi pranayama*, everyone exhale together</li></ul></li><li>Inhale raise your arms, shoulders heavy, hands light</li><li>Exhale, strong legs, keep the heart lifted as you fold forward</li></ul>

- Inhale lift your chest and broaden your shoulders, gaze up
- Exhale, step back to Rod, lower here if you want
- Inhaling roll over your feet to Upward Dog, strong legs
- Exhaling Downward Dog - at the end of your exhalation, bend your knees, look to your hands
- Inhale step your feet to your hands
- Exhale drop your sit bones into *Utkatasana*/the power posture
- Inhale, arms up in front, follow them with your gaze
    - Work *Utkatasana* for 5 breaths
    - Lightly hold the knees together
    - Heels ground, sit down deeply
    - Arms straight, work them back towards your ears
    - Work your torso toward being upright, chin lifted
- Exhale lower your arms down past your heart centre and fold forward
- Inhale lift your heart and broaden your collarbones
- Exhale step to Rod, lower if you wish
- Inhale pull your chest through to Upward Dog
- Exhale buttocks high to Downward Dog
- Inhale, up on your toes and step the right foot up
- Exhale replace the back heel at 45 degrees
- Inhale come up, adjust your stance if needed
- Exhale square your shoulders and hips
- Inhale shoulders down, raise your arms and gaze to your thumbs
    - Hold *Virabhadrasana*, the warrior posture for 5 breaths
    - Work both legs strongly, the right knee above the ankle, the left leg straight
    - Work the right hip back, the left hip forward to square your hips
    - Lift the pelvic floor, brace the lower abdomen
    - Shoulders down, neck long, chin lifting
    - Lower your gaze
- Inhale come up to change sides, arms stay up if you can or lower them shoulder height
- Exhaling, adjust your feet, arms up, gaze to your thumbs
    - Breathe fully feeling your chest move, listen to your breath
    - Bend deeply into the front leg, widen your stance if necessary
    - Extend out through your back leg ground down through the heel
    - Square your hips, the left hip works back, the right forward
    - Draw your shoulders down, lift your chin, gaze softly

[Do with, face-on]
- Inhale, now exhaling lower your arms down over your feet, open your hips and shoulders
- Open your back foot, widen your stance slightly, gaze to your left hand
    - Work *Virabhadrasana B* for 5 breaths
    - Your knee is exactly above your ankle and not beyond it
    - Work the knee back to open your hips
    - Keep equal grounding in both feet, especially the little toe side of your straight leg
    - Sit down with your buttocks, sit up with your trunk
- Inhale come up and swivel your feet to change sides
- Exhaling, bend the right knee to above your ankle, gaze to the right hand
    - Sit down deeply and keep a sense of buoyancy under your hips

	<ul><li>○ Both legs work strongly, the four corners of the feet grounding</li><li>○ Lift the pelvic floor, brace your lower belly</li><li>○ Breath fully into your chest, the ribs floating as you breath</li><li>○ Shoulders down, the front and back of the heart open</li></ul><ul><li>Inhaling turn to face your right foot, (come up onto the toes of the back foot)</li><li>Exhale hands to the floor either side of your front foot, step back to Rod</li><li>Inhale strong legs to Upward Dog</li><li>Exhale lead with the navel into Downward Dog</li><li>Bend your knees and come to sitting</li></ul>

Vinyasa - stepping

Overview	<ul><li>**Introduce stepping as an option in the *Vinyasa***</li><li>**Demonstrate the progression to stepping**</li><li>**Workshop problem areas before they attempt the move**</li><li>**Get them to practice this version in their own time**</li></ul>
Introduction	<ul><li>Up until now we've gone from standing to sitting using the same movements of our sun salutation, which in this context are called a *Vinyasa*.<ul><li>○ A *Vinyasa* is any sequential movement synchronised with breath<ul><li>■ [If not explained previously]</li></ul></li></ul></li><li>If you're doing well with that, I'll show you the next progression. It is only a slight variation on what you're already doing<ul><li>○ Remember you always have the option to stay doing the *Vinyasa* the way we are currently doing it<ul><li>■ I'll demonstrate first for you</li></ul></li></ul></li></ul>
Demonstrate side-on	<ul><li>The difference is that this time my knees do not come to the mat</li><li>From Downward Dog</li><li>Point your foot</li><li>Step it up</li><li>Second knee up</li><li>Cross the ankles and</li><li>Use your arms to pull you through<ul><li>○ If you can't get your legs through, knees to the floor</li><li>○ Flex the feet and push back to sitting</li></ul></li></ul>
Workshop	<ul><li>**Feet**<ul><li>○ It is really important to point your feet and keep them pointed as you come through</li><li>○ If you flex your feet you will be too high otherwise it will be more difficult to fit through your arms</li><li>○ **[Demonstrate side-on]**</li></ul></li></ul>

	- **Knees**
	  - With your ankles crossed keep your knees close together and
	  - Step far enough that your knees come between your hands
	  - Lift the knees toward your chest
	  - Try to roll yourself up into a little ball
	  - **[Demonstrate side-on]**
	
	- **Shoulders**
	  - Working the muscles of the whole of the upper body will help you to build the strength you will need for this movement
	    - Fingers spread wide, hands grounded
	    - Broaden your shoulder blades on your back to activate the muscles you need
	    - Draw the shoulder blades down your back and
	    - Pull yourself through using your arms
	    - **[Demonstrate side-on]**
	- **Alternative**
	  - If you aren't able to get your legs through your arms
	    - Place your knees to the floor
	    - Point your feet out to the sides and
	    - Gently push yourself back onto your buttocks
	    - **[Demonstrate side-on]**
	- To revise, we need to point the feet, keep the knees close together and use our arms to pull us through
	  - Are you ready to try all that?

Do With / Watch Them	- Come back to Downward Dog - At the end of your exhalation, bend your knees and look to your thumbs - Keep breathing and - Point one foot, step your knee up between your hands - Point the other foot and draw it up behind the first - Keep the knees close together - Shoulders broad, shoulder blades down and pull your legs through - If you don't make it, knees down, feet flexed and gently push back onto your buttocks - Play with that a couple more times in your own time

Week 5

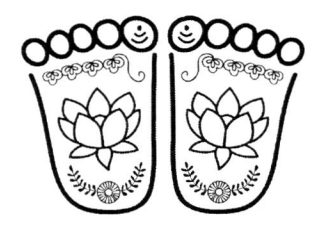

WEEK 5 • Strength & Endurance

Overview	• Revise lowering down in *Surya Namaskara*
	   o Lead through 3 *Surya Namaskara A*
	• **Teach hopping back & up in the sun salutations**
	   o Lead through 2 more *Surya Namaskara A*
	   o Lead through 3 *Surya Namaskara B*
	• **Teach hopping into the standing postures**
	• **Lead through the standing postures already taught**
	• **Revise *Parshvottanasana***
	• **Revise *UHP* preparation**
	• **Revise the Warrior Sequence**
	• **Teach *Dandasana* & *Pashimottanasana A & B***
	• **Teach *Purvottanasana***
	• **Teach a half *Vinyasa* (Stepping back & up)**
	• **Teach *Janu Shirshasana A & B***
	
	NOTE:
	• The C version for *Pashimottanasana* is not taught in this beginners program

Hopping in Sun Salutations	

Overview	• **Warm up with 3 *Surya Namaskara A***
	• **Introduce the concept of hopping in the *Surya Namaskara*s**
	• **Demonstrate hopping back & hopping up**
	• **Workshop hopping back and hopping up separately before they attempt them**
	   o Let them practice a few in their own time
	• **Give hopping as an option in the sun salutations**
	   o Lead through 2 more *Surya Namaskara A*
	   o Lead through 3 *Surya Namaskara B*

Introduction	• Traditionally, in *Ashtanga Yoga* instead of stepping back into our Rod with one foot at a time, we hop both feet back together, at the same time
	   o This builds strength and co-ordination
	• However, if you find it too strenuous, stay with stepping your feet back
	
	• Similarly, from Downward Dog we also bring both feet at the same time back towards the hands with a hop.
	• Again, if you find this too strenuous stay with stepping your feet up
	   o I'll show you how it's done

Demonstrate side-on	- **From *Trini***
	  o Exhale, hop back into Rod
	  o Inhale Upward Dog
	  o Exhale
	  o From Downward Dog
	  o Inhale, hop up

Workshop Hopping Back	- **Landing Lightly**
	  o To land lightly you need to keep as much weight as you can in your hands
	    - With your fingers spread wide
	    - Especially focus on keeping weight at the base of your fingers
	    - The shoulders must remain above the wrists
	  o If not you will land heavy on your feet
	    - **[Demonstrate the wrong way]**
	  o Try to land in a flat, strong Rod
	  o Keep your low belly firm when you land
	    - **[Demonstrate the right way]**

Do With / Watch Them	- Let's do one together
	- Everyone in a forward bend
	- Keep your shoulders over your wrists
	- Inhale lift your heart
	  o Bend your knees
	  o Keep the weight in your hands
	- Exhale, hop both feet back into a long, strong Rod
	- Come to your knees

Workshop Hopping Up	- **Buttocks high**
	  o When you hop up from Downward Dog it is important to keep your buttocks high
	    - Otherwise you'll land in a squat, which places a lot of stress on the knees
	    - **[Demonstrate dropping the buttocks and landing in a squat]**
	  o You keep your buttock high by not bending the knees too deeply
	    - **[Demonstrate hopping up with the buttocks high]**
	
	- **Using the arms**
	  o Using your arms will make the movement easier
	  o With our hands grounded, so they don't move, we pull our feet up to our hands
	
	- **Control**
	  o Keeping the lower ribs tucked into the waist will help you engage your abdominal muscles to give you more strength and control in this movement

	- **Gaze Position**
- Placing your gaze between your thumbs will help you to land in the right position
- If your gaze is too far towards your feet you will tend to land short of your hands or if it is too far forward of your hands you may travel too far forward
- Let's have a try
Do With / Watch Them	- From Downward Dog
- Tuck in your lower ribs
- At the end of your exhalation
- Bend your knees and look up between your hands
- Inhale, keep the buttocks high and
- Pull your feet up to your hands

- In your own time practice a few of these, playing with
    - Keeping the weight at the base of your fingers when you jump back
    - Using your arms to pull you up and
    - Keeping the buttocks high when you hop up

- If you feel comfortable with that, in the following sun salutations, substitute stepping with hopping. I'll remind you when |

Hopping in Standing Postures

Overview	- **Demonstrate**
- **Do it with them**
- **Watch & listen to them do it**
Introduction	- Similarly, as we did in the sun salutations, we can progress on in the standing postures by hopping both feet at the same time into and out of the standing postures
- Watch me, I'll show you how
Demonstrate face-on	**Jump Feet to Hip-width**
- Bending your knees to take off and
- Bend your knees to land
- It is important to bend the knees to give you height and momentum
- It is also very important to bend the knees on landing to cushion the impact
- Additionally, try to land on the balls of your toes, the heels follow
- Let's try that together

Do With/ Watch Them	• Inhale, bend your knees, hop up • Exhaling, land with bent knees • **[Listen to their landing]** • That sounds more like a herd of elephants than a class of yogis! • Let's try that again, please be gentle on the floor!

Dandasana	drishti: **toes**
Overview	• **Introduce *Dandasana*** • **Demonstrate** • **Do it with and watch them do the posture** • **Workshop any areas that need it** **NOTE:** • *Dandasana* is so simple it should not require that students do it twice • If you do the posture with them, face the class so you can watch them at the same time • Very stiff students may need to sit on the edge of a blanket
Introduction	• This is the first of the seated postures of the primary series in Ashtanga Yoga • It is called *Dandasana*, 'the staff' • *Dandasana* is like a seated *Samasthiti* ◦ All the same principles apply except that we are seated

Demonstrate side-on	• From the *Vinyasa*
	• Straighten your legs out
	• Arms extend down by your sides
	• Lift your heart, spine tall, long neck
	   ◦ Hold *Dandasana* for 5 breaths
	      ▪ Let's see you do it

Do With/ Watch Them	• Sit upright onto your sit bones and feel them heavy towards the floor • If you need, bend the knees to ensure that your low back does not round • Extend out through the base of your toes and heels • Maintain strong legs • Lightly ground your hands beside your hips and lift your heart • Keep the back of the chest broad and open • The heart area floats up and open in front • Gaze softly down towards your nose • Lengthen your spine and neck and lightly drop the chin • Breathe into all four areas of your chest • Listen to the sound of your breath

| Workshop

Demonstrate side-on | - **Low Back**
  - Sit upright onto your sit bones
  - Try to maintain some curve in your low back
    - If you can't, bend the knees as much as you need to, to feel your pelvis slightly tilt forward

- **Feet**
  - Extend out through the base of your toes and heels as you do in *Samasthiti*
    - As there is no floor to stop your feet, they will appear slightly pointed
    - Do not flex the feet back towards you

- **Arms**
  - If your arms are not long enough to ground your hands just reach them down towards the floor
  - If your arms are very long bend your elbows
  - The hands are placed in line with your hips
  - Without moving your hands, use a light swiping back action to draw your chest forward |

Pashimottanasana A & B   drishti: **toes**

Overview	- **Introduce *Pashimottanasana*** - **Demonstrate** - **Watch them do the posture** NOTE: - *Pashimottanasana* is simple enough that you do not need to do it with them - Very stiff students may need sit up on the edge of a blanket - This beginners program does not include *Pashimottanasana C*

Introduction	- In our second sitting posture we fold forward at the hips just as we did when we were standing
	- Again here we have a couple of variations on how we hold the feet
	- This posture is called *Pashimottanasana*, which means 'intense western stretch'
	  - The back of the body is referred to as the west and the front of the body the east, as traditionally, *Ashtanga Yoga* is practised facing the rising sun
	  - Watch me first

Demonstrate side-on
 	
A
 	
B
	[Demonstrate with knees bent, then straight]
	• From *Dandasana*
	• Bend your knees
	• Exhaling, fold forward, pick up the big toes
	• Inhale, lift your heart
	• Exhale, fold forward
	   o 5 breaths, belly on thighs, work toward straightening the legs
	• Inhale, lift up
	• Exhale hold the outside of your feet
	• Inhale lift
	• Exhale forward
	   o 5 breaths
	• Inhale up
	• Exhale release
	   o Now let me see you do it

Do With/ Watch Them	• Sitting upright in *Dandasana*
	• Bend the knees and reach forward to pick up your big toes
	   o Take the same grip as when we were standing
	• Inhale, lift your heart and
	• Exhale, fold forward, gazing to your toes
	• Keeping your belly kissing your thighs, work toward straightening your legs, until you feel some stretch in the back of your legs
	• Extend out through the four corners of your feet
	• Do not pull on your poor toes
	• Spread your sit bones wide
	• Work a gentle stretch into the back of your thighs
	• Continue to draw your shoulders down away from your ears
	• Lengthen through your entire spine
	• Drop the chin to keep your throat soft
	• Lengthen the back of your neck
	
	B
	• Inhale, lift your heart and hold the outside edges of your feet
	• Exhale here
	• Inhale, lift our of your hips
	• Exhale, fold forward
	   o [Repeat another 5 breaths with some of the same and other appropriate instructions]

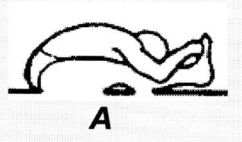

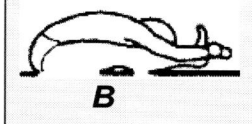

Purvottanasana   drishti: nose

Overview	• **Introduce *Purvottanasana*** • **Demonstrate arms only** • **Demonstrate arms & legs only** • **Demonstrate arms, legs & neck together, the complete posture** o Do it with them & watch them do each section

	NOTE: • Be sure to check that students have no neck problem before they attempt to take their head back • You will need to diligently check students' hand placement • Breaths will be shorter as the posture is strenuous

Introduction	• Our next posture counteracts the last posture
	• It is called *Purvottanasana* or 'intense eastern stretch'
	   o As we stretch the front of our body
	• We'll break it down into what we do with the arms first and then the legs to make it easier
	   o Watch me first

Demonstrate side-on ARMS	**Arms** • We place our hands one hands-length back away from our hips • The fingers point back towards you • Straighten your arms and • Inhaling lift your chest as high as possible • Exhale come down o Let's try that together
Do With / Watch Them	**[Walk around to check hand position]** • Hands one hands-length back away from your hips • The fingers point back towards you • Straighten your arms and keeping them straight • Inhale lift your chest as high as possible • Exhale and relax

Demonstrate side-on ADD ON LEGS	**Add on Legs**
	• Now we'll add on the legs
	   o Hands in position - one hands-length away from your hips
	   o Fingers point to the feet
	   o Straight arms
	   o Lift your chest high
	   o Chin to chest
	   o Legs strong, straight, knees together
	      ▪ Heels press down into the mat
	      ▪ Feet pointed
	   o Inhale hips up
	   o Exhale come down
	      ▪ Your turn

Do With / Watch Them	• To get up easily it is really important to work the legs correctly
	• So let's add that action with the legs onto the arms
	   o Hands back in position - one hands-length from the hips
	   o Fingers pointing in the direction of your feet
	   o Straighten your arms
	   o Lift your chest as high as possible
	   o Chin to the chest

	<ul><li>o Legs strong and straight</li><li>o Press the back of your heels down into the mat</li><li>o Inhale lift your hips<ul><li>▪ Work your toes towards the floor</li><li>▪ Drag your feet toward your hands</li><li>▪ Keep your chin to your chest</li><li>▪ Lightly squeeze your legs together</li></ul></li><li>o Exhale lower your hips to the mat</li></ul>
Demonstrate side-on HEAD POSITION **Full Posture**	**Head Position / Full Posture** <ul><li>Now I'll show you the full posture with the final head position</li><li>If you do not have a neck problem you can take your head back in this posture<ul><li>o The head just hangs back</li></ul></li><li>There is no 'half-way' position with the head in this posture<ul><li>o The head is either held up, chin on chest, or it hangs back</li><li>o Holding the head half-way puts a lot of stress on the neck muscles</li><li>o If after taking your head back, you find it uncomfortable, come down, hips first, and then go back into the posture with your chin on your chest. Do not change your head position in the posture<ul><li>▪ I'll show you the complete posture</li></ul></li><li>o Hands into position</li><li>o Arms straight</li><li>o Lift the heart high</li><li>o Ground the heels, feet pointed</li><li>o Inhale, lift the hips</li><li>o Exhale, chin on the chest OR</li><li>o Head hands back<ul><li>▪ [1 or 2 two breaths]</li></ul></li><li>o Exhale hips down first, head last<ul><li>▪ Your turn</li></ul></li></ul></li></ul>
Do With / Watch Them	<ul><li>Position your hands<ul><li>o One hands length back away from your hips</li><li>o The fingers point back towards your feet</li></ul></li><li>Straighten your arms</li><li>Inhale lift your chest as high as you can</li><li>Strong legs, lifting your kneecaps</li><li>Press the back of your heels down into the mat, point your feet</li><li>Inhale lift your hips</li><li>Exhale, keep your chin on your chest or take your head back and let it hang there<ul><li>o Gaze softly towards the tip of your nose</li><li>o Keep the heels pressing down</li><li>o Work the feet towards the floor</li><li>o Ground your hands strongly and</li><li>o Continue to lift the chest high</li></ul></li><li>Exhale, lower the hips, then head, and come out of the posture</li></ul>

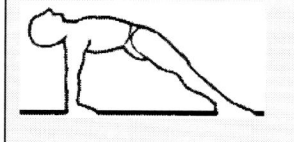

Vinyasa – Stepping Back	

Overview	- Introduce *Vinyasa* to come out of a posture - Demonstrate *Vinyasa* - Do it with them - Watch them do it - Give the alternative (Side-saddle) for those who find it too challenging **NOTE:** - In this beginners program a *vinyasa* is only given between every second sitting posture
Introduction	- Just as we have connecting movements or *Vinyasa* to get us from standing to sitting, we also use these same movements to connect one sitting posture to the next - As you're just starting we'll only do a *Vinyasa* between every second sitting posture - I'll show you how it's done

Demonstrate side-on	**Easy Option**
	- Cross the ankles and tuck the feet under, in close to your buttocks
	  - You will need to use your hands to tuck the feet under
	- Place your hands shoulder width just in front of your knees
	- Lean your weight forward into your hands
	- Exhaling, step back into your Rod
	- Inhale Upward Dog
	- Exhale Downward Dog
	- Inhale step back through to sitting
	
	Building Strength
	- If you would like a bigger challenge
	  - Cross the ankles
	  - Place your hands just forward of your buttocks
	  - Inhaling draw the feet through
	  - Exhale step back to Rod
	  - Inhale Upward Dog
	  - Exhale Downward Dog
	  - Inhale step back through to sitting

Workshop	**Important Pointers**
	- As when we stepped up to come to sitting, it is also important here to:
	  - Bend the arms and create space under your armpits
	  - Draw the knees up toward your chest and
	  - Suck the feet up toward your abdomen
	- The action of the shoulders is also the same
	  - Fingers spread wide, hands grounded
	  - Spread the shoulder blades broad on your back
	  - Pull yourself through

	Alternative (Side-saddle)
	[For those students who cannot perform either variation]
	    ○ Swing both legs to one side
	    ○ Exhaling, step back to Rod

**Do With /
Watch Them**
	• Cross the ankles, tuck your feet in close to your buttocks
	• Hands are shoulder width, just forward of your knees
	• Lean your weight into your hands
	• Exhale, step back to Rod
	• Inhale Upward Dog
	• Exhale Downward Dog
	OR
	• Cross your ankles and tuck your feet up
	• Bend your elbows and make space under your armpits
	• Keep your shoulder blades down and onto the back of your chest
	• Draw your knees up to your chest
	• Suck your feet up towards your armpits
	• Ground your hands just in front of your hips
	• Inhale, lift and pull yourself through
	• If you don't make it
	    ○ Bring your hands forward of your knees
	    ○ And step back to Rod
	• [Talk through stepping back to sitting]

Janu Shirshasana A	*drishti:* **toes**
Overview	• **Introduce *Janu Shirshasana A*** • **Demonstrate** • **Workshop the knee action before they do the posture** • **Do it with them on one side** • **Watch them do it on the other side** • **Workshop anything necessary** **NOTE**: • The hips are not squared in *Janu Shirshasana* A and B • Very stiff students may need to sit up on the edge of a blanket • This posture is best demonstrated face-on
Introduction	• This posture helps to open the hips and stretches the low back • We'll learn an A and a B version ○ Watch me

Demonstrate face-on	- From *Dandasana*, our upright Rod
	  o Bend the right leg and take the knee out
	  o Work the knee back and square the shoulders
	  o Inhale, lift up
	  o Exhale, forward
	    ▪ 5 breaths
	  o Inhale, lift
	  o Exhale release the posture and change sides

Workshop	**Protect the Knee**
	- With any hip rotation exercise it is important to protect your knee as it is capable of very little rotation
	  o When you bend up your leg, close the knee joint until it is completely sealed
	  o Keep it closed as you take your knee out to the side
	  o Continue to work the knee back
	    ▪ The maximum knee position is 90 degrees
	  o Point your right foot and
	  o Work the sole of your foot up to the ceiling / to face you
	    ▪ This will help to rotate your hip/give the correct rotation in your hip

Do With / Watch Them	- Bend up the right knee and seal off the knee joint
	- Let your knee down to the side
	- Point your foot and work the sole up to face you
	- Now work your knee back to open your hips
	- Square your shoulders to the straight leg, hold the leg, shoulders down, lift your heart
	- Inhale, lift out of your hips
	- Exhale, tip the pelvis forward
	  o We work in the posture for 5 breaths
	  o Gaze up to your toes, keeping the back of your neck long
	  o Remember to breath into all 4 areas of your chest, listening to your breath
	  o Both legs are working, the right knee back, the left leg strong
	  o Keep your lower abdomen firm, try to recreate the curve in your low back
	- Inhale, lift the chest
	- Exhale, release the posture and straighten the right leg
	- Other side

Workshop	**Torso Position** - **[Demonstrate face or side-on]** - Remember to square off your shoulders and torso - Keep your heart lifted - Then fold forward trying to keep the natural curve in your low back - The gaze is lifted to the toes

| | **Extended Leg**
• **[Demonstrate side-on]**
• Don't forget to work your straight leg by grounding out through the base of your toes and heels
• Keep the kneecaps lifted |

Janu Shirshasana B   drishti: toes

Overview	• **Introduce *Janu Shirshasana B*** • **Demonstrate** • **Workshop foot & knee positions before they do the posture** • **Walk around and watch them do it** **NOTE**: • This posture is best demonstrated face-on • Do not do *Janu Shirshasana B* with them as it is important to watch them and help them with the correct leg position • Screen the class for anyone who has had knee surgery - extreme flexion is unsuitable for students with surgical pins in their knees • For some students this posture will be uncomfortable on the front of their foot where it contacts the floor. You may get them to spread out a blanket so their foot is cushioned – unless you like a more austere bed-of-nails approach!
Intro	• So this is the B version of *Janusirsasana* o You'll soon work out why!

Demonstrate face-on	• Again from *Dandasana*
	• Inhaling bend the right knee and take it out to the side
	   o This time flex the foot and
	   o The knee comes in a little
	   o Inhale, lift the hips and come forward to sit on the heel
	      ▪ The heel fits in the crease of your buttocks/between the cheeks of your buttocks
	• Again square the torso to the straight leg
	• Inhaling, hold the leg, lift up
	• Exhale fold forward
	   o 5 breaths here
	• Inhale, lift up
	• Exhale release the posture and change sides

Workshop	**Important** • If you have had knee surgery and especially have surgical pins in your knee this posture is unsuitable for you o Instead, you can place your foot in the position but do not lift up and sit on the heel

	Foot
	• **[Demonstrate face-on]**
	• So let's look at the different foot position more closely
	    o This time the foot is flexed (opposite to pointed) to rest along the inside of the opposite thigh
	        ▪ This means the knee will come in about 5 degrees from where it was in *Janusirsasana A*/ the first version
	    o You may need adjust your foot position when you sit on the heel to find a comfortable position
	        ▪ Yes! Eventually this does feel comfortable
	
	Knee
	• **[Demonstrate face-on]**
	• When you lift your hips and move forward to sit on your heel
	• Ensure that you come forward far enough
	• So that your thigh is completely over the top of your calf
	    o This is important to protect your knee
	• If this posture feels uncomfortable on your knee, try bringing the knee further forward
	    o If it is still uncomfortable, keep the foot in position but do not lift up and sit on the heel
	• Let's try that
	• I'll walk around to check you're in the right position

Do With / Watch Them	• Bend up your right knee and close off the knee joint
	• Let your knee down to the side
	• Place your flexed foot along the inside of your left thigh
	• With an inhalation lift up your hips and move forward to sit on your right heel
	    o Your heel sits in the crease of your buttocks
	    o Adjust the position of your foot as you need to get comfortable
	• Look down at your right leg and check that your thigh covers your calf
	• Square off your shoulders and torso to the left straight leg
	• Inhale, holding the leg, lift your heart
	• Exhale, tip the pelvis forward
	    o We'll work here for 5 breaths
	    o Gaze up to your toes, draw your shoulders down, keep the back of your neck long
	    o Breath fully and deeply, listening to the *ujjayi* sound
	    o Both legs remain active
	    o Draw up from the base of your spine and draw your navel in towards your low back
	• Inhale, lift the chest high
	• Exhale, release the posture, straighten your right leg and we'll do the other side
	    o [Repeat same or other suitable instructions for the left side]

Week 6

WEEK 6 • The Flow of the Practice

Class Overview	• **Revise hopping in the sun salutations**
	    ○ Lead through 5 *Surya Namaskara A*
	    ○ Lead through 3 *Surya Namaskara B*
	• **Revise hopping into the standing postures**
	• **Lead through all the standing postures and Warrior sequence**
	• **Revise *Dandasana* & *Pashimottanasana* A & B**
	• **Revise *Purvottanasana***
	• **Teach half *Vinyasa* (Hopping)**
	• **Revise *Janu Shirshasana* A & B**
	• **Teach *Marichyasana* A & C**
	• **Teach *Navasana***
	• **Lead through the sitting finishing postures & *Shavasana***
	
	NOTE:
	• Attempt to give students a taste of the 'flow' and 'heat' of Ashtanga Yoga - if possible talk them through the postures they know without any pauses
	• Encourage students to continue onto the next level class/ course

REVISION: Hopping in Sun Salutations	

Overview	• **Revise hopping back and up**
	    ○ **Give the option to insert into the sun salutations**
	    ○ **Lead them through 5 *Surya Namaskara A***
	    ○ **Lead them through 3 *Surya Namaskara B***

Introduction & Demonstration side-on	• You may remember last week how you learnt another way to get into the Rod, where we hopped the feet back together
	    ○ I'll show you again
	    ○ From the third position in the sun salutation we hop our feet back together
	    ○ And again from our Downward Dog you can hop both feet back at the same time
	• **Hopping Back**
	    ○ Try to land lightly by keeping the weight in your hands
	        ▪ Especially at the base of your fingers
	    ○ And try to land in a flat, strong Rod
	• **Hopping Up**
	    ○ Remember it is important to keep your buttocks high so you don't land in a squat
	        ▪ Gaze up between your thumbs
	        ▪ And don't forget to use your arms
	            - Pull your feet up to our hands
	• Remember, if you find this too strenuous stay with stepping your feet back and up
	    • Or insert the hopping in only some of the sun salutations

TALK-THROUGH: *Surya Namaskara A*

Overview	- **Talk students through without stopping**
	  - Should they really need a break, do this in *Samasthiti* with instruction
	
	- **If something looks unsound or unsafe**
	  - First attempt to give instructions and use touch to correct
	    - If this does not work, stop and workshop that area
	
	- **Keep an even, rhythmic pace**
	  - You will need to vary the rate at which you speak: more quickly to include a long instruction and slow down your speech if the next instruction is shorter
	    - Aim to keep their breath at the same rate
	
	- **Downward Dog**
	  - Start with the most important instructions
	  - Cover the entire posture over the five breaths
	  - Have a program for each Downward Dog or overall during the sun salutations
	    - Start with the feet or hands and work over the body
	    - Begin specific and get more generalised, etc
	  - The instructions given here are for one whole breath (inhale + exhale)
	  - *Drishti* for beginners is between the knees
	
	- **There are a multitude of possible instructions for *Surya Namaskara***
	  - The objective is to cover all the important aspects of the posture
	  - To give a variety of instructions to give students every possibility to understand how to do the posture safely and effectively
	  - Instructions from learning *Samasthiti* or the other teaching phases of the sun salutations may be used
	    - Below are some more examples

Samasthiti	- Ground the four corners of your feet, suctioning the insteps - Grow your legs tall and strong - Continue a sensation of lifting from you feet, up your legs and over into your pelvis, checking that your bandhas are engaged - Drop the sit bones and lift your pelvic floor - Buttocks firm but not clenched, brace your lower abdomen, - Lift your heart, open the back of your chest and breathe in all directions, feel your ribs move/float as you breathe - Loop your shoulders back and down, keeping the shoulder blades broad on your back - Lightly extend through your arms and fingers - Lengthen your neck, your shoulders and ears backing away from each other - Gently draw your ears back in line with your shoulders - Drop the chin slightly to soften your throat/front of your neck

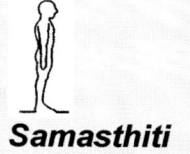

	- Soften your face and gaze to the floor in front of you - Check that your posture feels light and balanced - Tune into the sound of your breath - Ready for *Surya Namaskara A*, everyone exhale together
Ekam 1	- Inhale, keep your shoulders low and raise your arms, gaze up - Inhale, shoulders heavy, light arms, palms meet, gaze to the thumbs - Inhale, turn your palms up, shoulders down, reach your arms up above your head, look up - Inhale, raise your arms, lifting your chin at the same rate as your arms and gaze up - Inhale, shoulders down, arms up, lift your chin to gaze to your thumbs
Dve 2	- Exhale, keep the heart lifted, take the long way down, drop your head - Exhale, ground your feet, strong legs, tip your hips forward, belly touches the thighs - Exhale, fold forward, splay your sit bones, belly kissing the thighs - Exhale, strong legs, low belly firm, fold forward, drop your head - Exhale, strong legs, fold forward at the hips, drop your head - Exhale, fold forward, work to keep the curve in your low back
Trini 3	- Inhale, fingers touch the floor, lift your heart, your head and your gaze - Inhale, lift your chest, shoulders down, back of the neck long - Inhale, lift your chest, broaden your shoulders, look up - Inhale, lift your heart, widen your collarbones, look up - Inhale, heart, head and gaze lift, shoulders down
Chatvari 4	- Exhale, step or hop back into the Rod, low belly strong - Exhale, fingers spread wide, weight in the hands, step or hop back - Exhale, back to Rod, lower here, elbows hug your torso - Exhale, back and lower into Rod, push out through the heels - Exhale, Rod, draw the chest forward between your hands - Exhale, Rod, pinch your shoulder blades together on your back - Exhale, Rod, drop your chin, face parallel to the floor - Exhale, Rod, push out through the heels, chest draws forward
Pancha 5	- Inhale, roll over your toes to Upward Dog, draw your chest forward - Inhale to Upward Dog, use your arms to draw you forward - Inhale, Upward Dog, strong legs, draw the heart forward, look up - Inhale, strong legs, brace your low belly, lift the chin, look up Inhale, - Inhale, press the top of your feet into the mat, gaze upward - Inhale, spread the fingers, roll the shoulder back and down - Inhale, use you feet as brakes, the arms to traction your spine

Shat 6	• Exhale, push off your hands into Downward Dog
	• Exhale, lift from your navel into Downward Dog
	• Exhale, buttocks high into Downward Dog
	• Exhale, buttocks up, head down, Downward Dog
	    o Drop your heels, check your feet are straight and hip-width apart
	    o Strong legs, lift your kneecaps, gaze between the knees
	    o Splay your sit bones wide and work them to the ceiling
	    o Tip the pelvis forward, try to recreate the curve in your low back
	    o Elongate the whole of your spine, including your neck
	    o Use the weight of your head to lengthen your neck
	    o Back of the head in line with the rest of your spine
	    o Drop your chin to keep the front of the neck soft
	    o Soften the lowest ribs back into your abdomen
	    o Draw your shoulder blades back up toward the hips
	    o Breathe into the space between your shoulder blades
	    o Feel the arms working back into your shoulder joints
	    o Strong arms, feel them propping you up
	    o Work your shoulders down away from your ears
	    o Crown of the head works forward towards your hands
	    o Spread your fingers, middle finger points straight ahead
	    o Check that the base of your fingers and thumb touch the mat
	    o Ground through the base of your thumb and fingers
	    o Ground your hands, transfer your weight back toward your feet
	    o Soften your face and gaze softly between your knees
	    o Breathe fully, feel your ribs move with the breath
	    o Breathe into the front, sides and back of your chest
	    o Feel your ribs float as you breathe
	    o Listen to the sound of your breath
	    o Heels heavy, strong legs, hands grounding, strong arms
	    o Imagine you're a tent, your hands and feet the pegs grounding, your hips the highest point
	    o Feel the strength and support of your limbs as you elongate your spine
	    o Strong arms and legs, release your spine
	• At the end of your exhalation, bend your knees, look to your hands

Sapta 7	• Inhale, step or hop your feet up, lift your heart, head and gaze • Inhale pull the feet up between your hands, look up • Inhale, use your arms to step or hop up, keep lifting, look up • Inhale, keep the buttocks high as you step or hop the feet up
Ashtau 8	• Exhale, fold forward, splay your sit bones, belly kissing the thighs • Exhale, fold forward, work towards straightening the legs • Exhale, forward, low belly firm, drop your head • Exhale, forward, strong legs, long spine and neck • Exhale, forward, a gentle stretch in the back of your legs

Nava 9	• Inhale, keep your shoulders low and raise your arms, gaze up • Inhale, shoulders heavy, light arms, palms together, look to your thumbs • Inhale, turn your palms up, shoulders down, reach your arms up above your head, look up • Inhale, raise your arms, lifting your chin at the same rate as your arms and gaze up • Inhale, shoulders down, arms up, lift your chin to gaze to your thumbs
Samasthiti	• Exhale, back to *Samasthiti* • Exhale, *Samasthiti*, the equal-standing posture • Exhale, *Samasthiti*, gaze softly downward

TALK-THROUGH:	***Surya Namaskara B***

Overview	• **See overview for *Surya Namaskara A***
	
	NOTE:
	• The extra breath given to beginners to enter *Virabhadrasana* should be removed by their last class to prepare them for the next level of classes
	   o Replace it with the 'Cheats Version' of getting into *Virabhadrasana*:
	       ▪ Use the end of the exhalation of Downward Dog to step their foot up between the hands

Samasthiti	• *Surya Namaskara B* • Everyone exhale together
Ekam 1	• Inhale, drop your sit bones, knees together, arm straight up in front, gaze to your thumbs • Inhale, deeply bend your knees, shoulders down raise your arms up the centre, gaze up • Inhale, squat low, shoulders heavy, straight arms, palms together, follow your thumbs • Inhale, • Inhale, as you lower your buttocks, raise your arms, lift your gaze to follow your thumbs • Inhale, drop the buttocks, shoulders down, arms up in front, gaze to your thumbs

Dve 2	• Exhale, keep the heart lifted, take the long way down, drop your head • Exhale, ground your feet, strong legs, tip your hips forward, belly touches the thighs • Exhale, fold forward, splay your sit bones, belly kissing the thighs • Exhale, strong legs, low belly firm, fold forward, drop your head • Exhale, draw up your kneecaps, fold forward, drop your head • Exhale, work your legs, fold forward, work to keep the curve in your low back
Trini 3	• Inhale, fingers touch the floor, lift your heart, your head and your gaze • Inhale, lift your chest, shoulders down, back of the neck long • Inhale, lift your chest, broaden your shoulders, look up • Inhale, lift your heart, widen your collarbones, look up • Inhale, heart, head and gaze lift, shoulders down
Chatvari 4	• Exhale, step or hop back into the Rod, low belly strong • Exhale, fingers spread wide, weight in the hands, step or hop back • Exhale, back to Rod, lower here, elbows hug your chest • Exhale, back and lower into Rod, push out through the heels • Exhale, Rod, draw the chest forward between your hands • Exhale, Rod, shoulder blades broad on your back • Exhale, Rod, drop your chin, face parallel to the floor • Exhale, Rod, lift your face and shoulder away from the floor
Pancha 5	• Inhale, roll over your toes to Upward Dog, draw your chest forward • Inhale to Upward Dog, use your arms to draw you forward • Inhale, Upward Dog, strong legs, draw the heart forward, look up • Inhale, strong legs, brace your low belly, lift the chin, look up Inhale, • Inhale, press the top of your feet into the mat, gaze upward • Inhale, spread the fingers, roll the shoulder back and down • Inhale, use you feet as brakes, the arms to traction your spine
Shat 6	• Exhale, lift from your navel into Downward Dog • Stay up high on your toes • **Cheat's Version** ○ Step the right foot up, ground the back foot at 45 degrees

Sapta 7	• **Extra Breath**
	    ○ Inhale, lift your torso, hands to your hips
	    ○ Exhale square your hips
	    ○ Inhale, raise the arms and gaze up to your thumbs
	• Inhale, raise the arms, shoulders down, look up to your thumbs

Ashtau 8	• Exhale, hands down, step back to Rod • Exhale, down and back to the Rod, push out through the heels • Exhale, down and back to Rod, pull your sternum/chest forward • Exhale, down to Rod, squeeze the shoulder blades together • Exhale, down to Rod, lower your chest between your hands • Exhale, down to Rod, face parallel to the floor
Nava 9	• Inhale roll over your toes to Upward Dog, strong legs • Inhale, Upward Dog, pull the chest forward • Inhale, Upward Dog, brake with your feet, pull your heart through • Inhale Upward Dog, strong legs, lift the kneecaps • Inhale, Upward Dog, shoulders back and down
Dasha 10	• Exhale buttocks up to Downward Dog, up on your toes • Exhale, push off your hands into Downward Dog, up on your toes • Exhale, push the buttock high into Downward Dog, up on your toes • **Cheat's Version** • Step the right foot up (between your hands), ground the back foot at 45 degrees

Ekadasha 11	• **Extra Breath**
	   ○ Inhale, lift your torso, hands to your hips
	   ○ Exhale square your hips
	   ○ Inhale, arms up, gaze up to the thumbs
	• Inhale, arms up, shoulders down, chin up to gaze to the thumbs

Dvadasha 12	• Exhale, Rod, squeeze the shoulder blades together • Exhale, Rod, lower your chest between your hands • Exhale, Rod, push out through the heels • Exhale, Rod, the heart draws forward • Exhale, Rod, face parallel to the floor
Trayodasha 13	• Inhale roll over your toes to Upward Dog, strong legs • Inhale, Upward Dog, pull the chest forward • Inhale, Upward Dog, brake with your feet, pull your heart through • Inhale, Upward Dog, pull the chest through • Inhale Upward Dog, strong legs, lift the kneecaps • Inhale, Upward Dog, shoulders back and down

Chaturdasha 14	• Exhale, push off your hands, buttocks high into Downward Dog
	• Exhale, buttocks high into Downward Dog
	• Exhale, butt up, head down, Downward Dog
	   ○ Drop your heels, check your feet are straight and hip-width apart
	   ○ Strong legs, lift your kneecaps, gaze between the knees
	   ○ Splay your sit bones wide and work them to the ceiling
	   ○ Tip the pelvis forward, try to recreate the curve in your low back
	   ○ Elongate the whole of your spine, including your neck

	<ul><li>○ Use the weight of your head to lengthen your neck</li><li>○ Back of the head in line with the rest of your spine</li><li>○ Drop your chin to keep the front of the neck soft</li><li>○ Soften the lowest ribs back into your abdomen</li><li>○ Draw your shoulder blades back up toward the hips</li><li>○ Breathe into the space between your shoulder blades</li><li>○ Feel the arms working back into your shoulder joints</li><li>○ Strong arms, feel them propping you up</li><li>○ Work your shoulders down away from your ears</li><li>○ Crown of the head works forward towards your hands</li><li>○ Spread your fingers, middle finger points straight ahead</li><li>○ Check that the base of your fingers and thumb touch the mat</li><li>○ Ground through the base of your thumb and fingers</li><li>○ Ground your hands, transfer your weight back toward your feet</li><li>○ Soften your face and gaze softly between your knees</li><li>○ Breathe fully, feel your ribs move with the breath</li><li>○ Breathe into the front, sides and back of your chest</li><li>○ Feel your ribs float as you breathe</li><li>○ Listen to the sound of your breath</li><li>○ Heels heavy, strong legs, hands grounding, strong arms</li><li>○ Imagine you're a tent, your hands and feet the pegs grounding, your hips the highest point</li><li>○ Feel the strength and support of your limbs as you elongate your spine</li><li>○ Strong arms and legs, release your spine</li><li>• At the end of your exhalation, bend your knees, look to your hands</li></ul>
Panchadasa 15	<ul><li>Inhale, step or hop your feet up, lift your heart, head and gaze</li><li>Inhale pull the feet up between your hands, look up</li><li>Inhale, use your arms to step or hop up, keep lifting, look up</li><li>Inhale, keep the buttocks high as you step or hop the feet up</li></ul>
Shodasha 16	<ul><li>Exhale, fold forward, splay your sit bones wide</li><li>Exhale, forward, your belly kissing your thighs</li><li>Exhale, fold forward, work towards straightening the legs</li><li>Exhale, draw your navel towards your spine as you fold forward</li><li>Exhale, low belly firm as you fold forward, drop your head</li><li>Exhale, strong legs, fold forward, long spine and neck</li></ul>
Saptadasha 17	<ul><li>Inhale, drop your sit bones, knees together, arm straight up in front, gaze to your thumbs</li><li>Inhale, deeply bend your knees, shoulders down, raise your arms up the centre, gaze up</li><li>Inhale, squat low, shoulders heavy, straight arms, palms together, follow your thumbs</li><li>Inhale, as you lower your buttocks, raise your arms, lift your gaze to follow your thumbs</li><li>Inhale, drop the buttocks, shoulders down, arms up in front, gaze to your thumbs</li></ul>

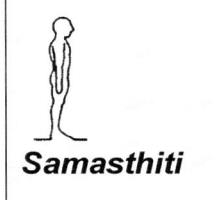

Samasthiti	• Exhale, back to *Samasthiti* • Exhale, *Samasthiti*, the equal-standing posture • Exhale, *Samasthiti*, gaze softly down

TALK-THROUGH:	***Padangustasana* to *UHP* Preparation**

Overview	• **Attempt to lead students through the standing postures with almost no breaks**
	  ○ This will depend on the talent of the group
	
	• **If any area really needs workshopping**
	  ○ Use this as a break
	
	• **You will not be doing the postures with the students but**
	  ○ You may need to assume some positions to refresh their memory or to spur them on, for example
	    ▪ The knee position in *Parshvakonasana*
	    ▪ The arm position in *Prasarita C*, etc
	
	• **Take extra breaths if necessary to get students correctly into any posture**
	
	• **Periodically allow them a few breaths in *Samasthiti* (with instructions) to recuperate and re-establish their breathing**
	
	• **Instructions for the 5 breaths in the *asana***
	  ○ Two complimentary instructions are given for each full breath (inhale+exhale) – these also may be used singularly
	  ○ Keep your breath counts to the same length of time (ie. If you use a long instruction on the inhale your exhale instruction should also be long or pause to allow for the extra time)
	  ○ Ensure that your instructions cover the important aspects of the entire posture
	  ○ Remember to include the *drishti*
	  ○ Try to vary your instructions from one side to the other of the same posture
	    ▪ Attempt to use different wording even if you are giving the same instruction
	  ○ Have a system, eg:
	    ▪ Start from the feet and work up or *vice versa*
	    ▪ Juxtaposition one instruction with its opposite
	    ▪ Give specific instructions on one side, more general instructions on the other, etc
	  ○ There are many ways to say the same thing. Those given below are some examples that do work.
	  ○ Remember that many of the instructions given in *Samasthiti* may be included in most other postures

Padangustasana	From *Samasthiti*
	• Inhale draw your hands up into *Namaste*
	• Exhale bend your knees and step or lightly hop your feet hip-width apart
	    ○ Hands to your hips
	• Inhale ground your feet and lift up out of your hips
	• Exhale, strong legs, fold forward
	• Inhale pick up your big toes, lift your heart
	• Exhale drop your head, gazing softly toward your nose
	    ○ Continue to breath into the front, side, back and top of the chest, listening to the *ujjayi* sound
	    ○ Check that the four corners of your feet ground evenly and your insteps lift away from the floor
	    ○ Keep your low abdomen close to your thighs and work towards straightening the legs a little more
	    ○ Continue to lift your pelvic floor and lightly brace the lower abdomen
	    ○ Your shoulders draw away from your ears, your neck and spine extending long
	• Inhale lift your heart

Pada Hastasana	• Exhale place your fingers under your feet
	    ○ Breath fully and return your *drishti* or gaze toward your nose
	    ○ As you lift your shoulders away from the floor, let the weight of your head traction/lengthen your spine
	    ○ The legs work strongly, the back releases
	        ▪ Imagine you're hanging over a fence where your legs become the fence, strong and supportive
	        ▪ Allow the whole of your back and spine lengthen and relax
	• Inhale lift your heart, your head and gaze
	• Exhale, stay forward/there, hands to your hips
	• Inhale come up to standing
	• Exhale, step or hop back to *Samasthiti*

Trikonasana	• Inhale hands to *Namaste*
	• Exhale step or lightly hop to your right, landing your feet about 1m wide
	• Hands shoulder height
	• Inhale open your right foot to 90 degrees and turn your left foot in slightly
	• Exhale strong, straight legs
	• Inhale look to your right foot, keep your arms above your legs and reach as far as you can over your right foot
	• Exhale place your hand down to your leg and look up to your left thumb
	    ○ Keep breathing, keeping your breath full and the chest moving
	    ○ As your ground the feet, lift the insteps, lift your kneecaps
	    ○ Check that your right knee is not locked-out but rather just a fraction bent
	    ○ Keep both shoulders down away from your ears
	    ○ Lengthen the back of your neck
	• Look back straight ahead and inhale come up

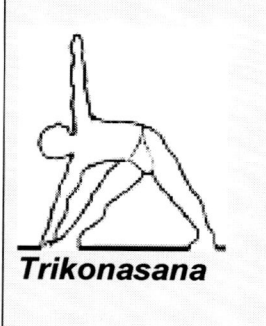

	<ul><li>Exhale change side, left foot 90 degrees, right foot in to about 5 degrees</li><li>Inhale, without leaning forward extend out over the left foot</li><li>Exhale left shoulder over left leg, right shoulder above the left, gaze up to your thumb<ul><li>5 breaths, strong legs, keep the kneecaps lifted</li><li>Draw up from the pelvic floor using *mullah bandha*</li><li>Keep the lower abdomen firm as you engage *uddiyana bandha*</li><li>Check that your neck is in line with the rest of your spine</li><li>Lengthen your neck and spine as you draw your shoulders down</li></ul></li><li>Inhale gaze back to the front and come up</li><li>Exhale, step or hop lightly back to *Samasthiti*</li></ul>
Ardha Parshvakonasana	<ul><li>Inhale hands on your chest in *Namaste*</li><li>Exhale step or lightly hop to your right, landing your feet wide</li><li>Hands land at shoulder height<ul><li>Open the right foot to 90 degrees, left foot turns in slightly</li><li>Now bend your right knee as deeply as you can - adjust your stance if necessary so your knee does not extend beyond your ankle</li><li>Keep your left leg strong and straight and work your right knee back to open your groins</li><li>Roll your arms to turn your palms up to the ceiling</li></ul></li><li>Inhale, keep the weight equal in both feet</li><li>Exhale, lower the right arm to rest your elbow on your knee</li><li>Inhale, look to the ceiling and raise your left arm up over your head<ul><li>We'll work the posture for 5 breaths</li><li>Check you still have weight in the left foot with the little toe side of your foot grounded/making contact with the mat</li><li>Both *bandhas* engaged, lifting the pelvic floor and the lower abdomen firm</li><li>Shoulders down away from your ears, left armpit works towards the floor, palm faces the floor</li><li>Lift your heart, back of the neck long, soft gaze</li></ul></li><li>Inhaling, push off your right foot and come upright</li><li>Exhale, change sides, right foot 90 degrees, left in slightly<ul><li>Keep weight in both feet and bend the left knee</li><li>Work your left knee back to open your groins</li><li>Roll your arms so your palms face the ceiling</li></ul></li><li>With an inhalation, lift out of your hips, lift your heart</li><li>Exhale lower the left elbow to your left thigh</li><li>Inhale reach the right arm up over your head, gaze to the ceiling<ul><li>Continue to push off the left foot to transfer weight back into the right foot</li><li>Do not collapse into the left hip but keep your hips buoyant away from the floor</li><li>Keep a lifting sensation from your insteps, up into your torso and along the entire length of your spine and neck</li><li>Work the right hand away from the right foot and your right foot away from your right hand</li><li>Keep the breath full and directed, moving the whole of your chest</li></ul></li><li>Inhaling, push off the left foot to bring yourself upright</li><li>Exhale square off your feet and step or hop back to *Samasthiti*</li></ul>

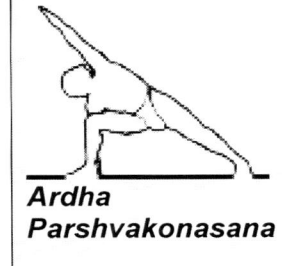

Prasarita Padottanasana

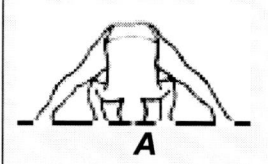

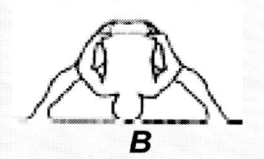

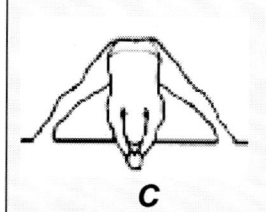

- Inhaling hands on your chest in *Namaste*
- Exhaling step or hop to your right, feet 1m apart, hands to hips

A version
- Look down to your feet and check that the outside edges of your feet are parallel - adjust your stance if you need to [only if necessary]
- Ground the four corners of your feet, lift your insteps, strong legs and engage your *bandhas*
- Inhale, lift your heart and look up
- Exhale, fold forward bending your knees as your need to, hands to the floor
- Inhale lift your chest, broaden your shoulders
- Exhale fold forward, hands to the floor between your feet
    - Check that your hands are straight and shoulder-width apart, spread your fingers wide
    - Lift your shoulders away from the floor and draw your shoulder blades up to your hips
    - Lengthen your spine and neck, keep them relaxed
    - Gaze toward the tip of your nose, keep your gaze soft
    - 5 full, directed breaths, notice your ribs move your breath
- Inhale lift your chest and head and look up
- Stay there/forward and exhaling place your hands on your hips
- Inhale, strong legs and come on up
- Exhale stay there

B version
- Inhale, keep the action in your feet and legs and extend your arms shoulder height
- Exhale hands to your hips
- Inhale lift up out of your feet
- Exhale fold forward
    - Keep your feet active and your legs strong
    - Continue the lift from your feet up your legs and up into your torso
    - Lift your pelvic floor and with your fingers, feel the lower belly firm
    - Release your spine and neck toward the floor
    - Actively lift your shoulders away from your ears and back up to your hips
- Inhale leading with your head, lift your torso and come upright
    - If this makes you light-headed take an extra breath to come up
- Exhale, hands stay on the hips

C version
- Inhaling, extend your arms out to shoulder height
- Exhaling, hands behind your back
    - Interlace your fingers
    - Roll your shoulder firmly back and
    - Work towards straightening your arms
    - Keeping your arms straight, breathe in and
- Exhale, fold forward
    - Maintain the position of your shoulders
    - Keep working the arms straight and let them release towards the floor
    - Bend your knees if you feel you low back round

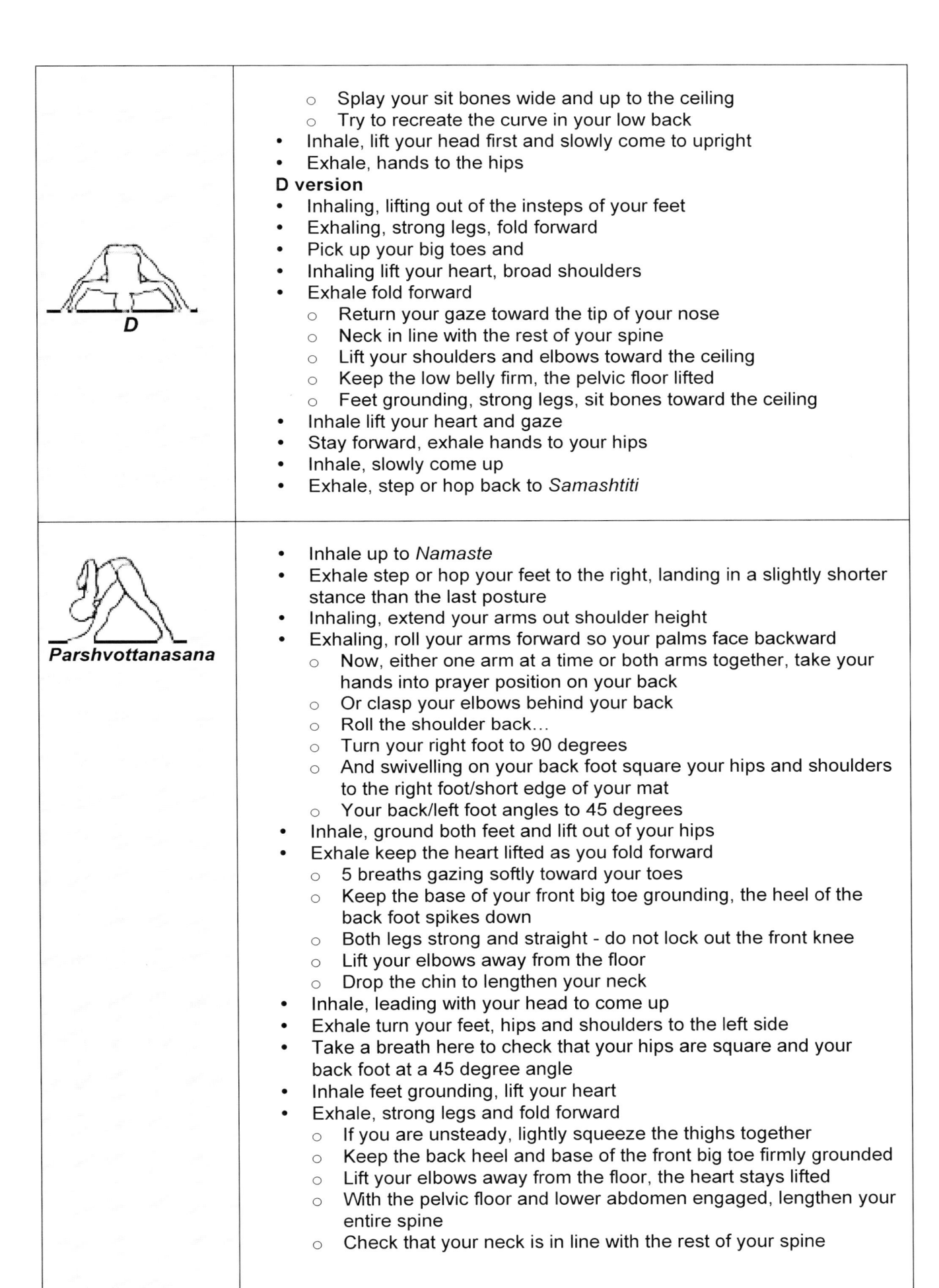

D	<ul><li>○ Splay your sit bones wide and up to the ceiling</li><li>○ Try to recreate the curve in your low back</li></ul>• Inhale, lift your head first and slowly come to upright • Exhale, hands to the hips **D version** • Inhaling, lifting out of the insteps of your feet • Exhaling, strong legs, fold forward • Pick up your big toes and • Inhaling lift your heart, broad shoulders • Exhale fold forward<ul><li>○ Return your gaze toward the tip of your nose</li><li>○ Neck in line with the rest of your spine</li><li>○ Lift your shoulders and elbows toward the ceiling</li><li>○ Keep the low belly firm, the pelvic floor lifted</li><li>○ Feet grounding, strong legs, sit bones toward the ceiling</li></ul>• Inhale lift your heart and gaze • Stay forward, exhale hands to your hips • Inhale, slowly come up • Exhale, step or hop back to *Samashtiti*
Parshvottanasana	• Inhale up to *Namaste* • Exhale step or hop your feet to the right, landing in a slightly shorter stance than the last posture • Inhaling, extend your arms out shoulder height • Exhaling, roll your arms forward so your palms face backward<ul><li>○ Now, either one arm at a time or both arms together, take your hands into prayer position on your back</li><li>○ Or clasp your elbows behind your back</li><li>○ Roll the shoulder back…</li><li>○ Turn your right foot to 90 degrees</li><li>○ And swivelling on your back foot square your hips and shoulders to the right foot/short edge of your mat</li><li>○ Your back/left foot angles to 45 degrees</li></ul>• Inhale, ground both feet and lift out of your hips • Exhale keep the heart lifted as you fold forward<ul><li>○ 5 breaths gazing softly toward your toes</li><li>○ Keep the base of your front big toe grounding, the heel of the back foot spikes down</li><li>○ Both legs strong and straight - do not lock out the front knee</li><li>○ Lift your elbows away from the floor</li><li>○ Drop the chin to lengthen your neck</li></ul>• Inhale, leading with your head to come up • Exhale turn your feet, hips and shoulders to the left side • Take a breath here to check that your hips are square and your back foot at a 45 degree angle • Inhale feet grounding, lift your heart • Exhale, strong legs and fold forward<ul><li>○ If you are unsteady, lightly squeeze the thighs together</li><li>○ Keep the back heel and base of the front big toe firmly grounded</li><li>○ Lift your elbows away from the floor, the heart stays lifted</li><li>○ With the pelvic floor and lower abdomen engaged, lengthen your entire spine</li><li>○ Check that your neck is in line with the rest of your spine</li></ul>

| | - Inhale, keep the heart lifted as you come up
- Exhale square off your feet, extend your arms out and step or hop back |
|---|---|
| **UHP Preparation** | **[Keep the breaths shorter in these positions]**
- Shift your weight into your left foot and
- Inhale bend your right knee and lift it to your chest with both hands
- Exhale place your left hand to your left hip
  - Lengthen through the inseam/inside of your standing leg grounding the inside corners of your foot
  - Keep your gaze steady to the floor or out in front of you
  - Keep your *bandhas* engaged, your low belly firm
  - Drop your shoulders and lengthen your neck
  - Keep breathing
- Inhale lift your knee a little higher and
- Exhale stay focused on your grounded foot and take the knee to the right
  - Only if you feel steady, turn your head and gaze to the opposite direction
  - Check that your torso remains upright
  - Lift out of your hips, heart lifted, chest open
  - Try to keep your breath full and directed
  - Stay focused…. and
- Inhaling, bring the knee and gaze back to centre
- Exhale both hands to your hips
- Inhaling keep your knee lifting/as high as you can and
- Exhale straighten your leg
  - Inside of the right foot grounding
  - Low belly braced
  - Heart lifted
  - Shoulders down
  - Soft gaze
- Exhaling lower your right leg
- Take an extra breath
- Shift your weight into your right foot and
- Inhaling lift your left knee, draw it to your chest with both hands
- Exhale place your right hand on your right hip
- [Use or modify any of the above or other appropriate instructions] |

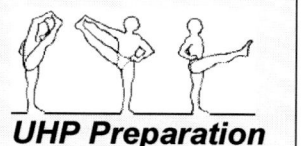

TALK-THROUGH: Warrior Sequence

| | - Standing in *Samasthiti*
  - Ground your feet, strong legs, *bandhas* engaged, open the front and back of your chest, shoulders down, front of the throat soft, soften your gaze
  - Establish you *ujjayi pranayama,* exhale together
- Inhale raise your arms, shoulders heavy, hands light
- Exhale, strong legs, keep the heart lifted as you fold forward
- Inhale lift your chest, broaden your shoulders |
|---|---|

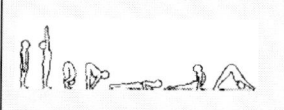

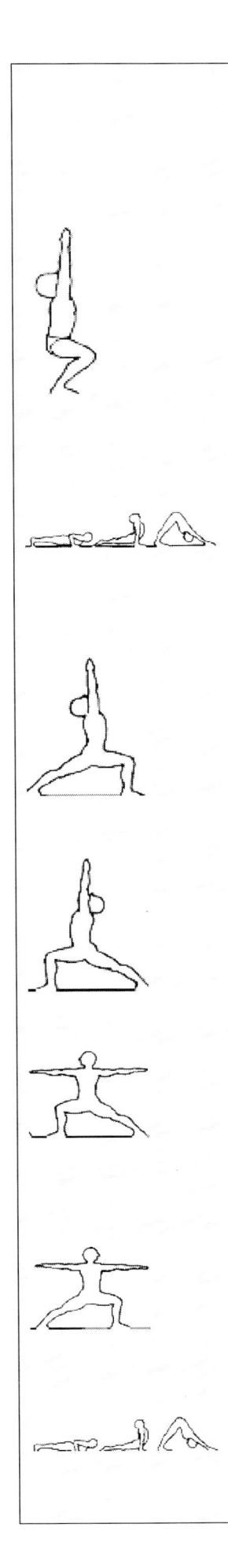

- Exhale, weight in your hands, step or hop your feet back, lower down
- Inhaling roll over your feet to Upward Dog, strong legs
- Exhaling Downward Dog - at the end of your exhalation, bend your knees, look to your hands
- Inhale, use your arms, step or hop your feet to your hands

[If necessary, do with them, side-on]
- Exhale drop your sit bones into *Utkatasana*/the power posture
- Inhale, palms together, arms up straight in front, follow them with your gaze
    - We work *Utkatasana* for 5 breaths
    - Lightly hold the knees together
    - Keep sitting down deeply
    - With your arms straight work them back towards your ears
    - Work your torso toward being upright, chin lifted
- Exhale lower your arms down the midline and fold forward
- Inhale lift your heart and widen your collarbones
- Exhale step or hop back to Rod, lower if you can
- Inhale pull your chest through to Upward Dog
- Exhale buttocks high to Downward Dog
- Inhale, come up on your toes and step the right foot up
- Exhale replace the back heel at 45 degrees
- Inhale come up, adjust your stance if needed
- Exhale square your hips
- Inhale shoulders down, palms up, raise your arms and gaze up to your thumbs
    - Hold *Virabhadrasana*, the warrior posture for 5 breaths
    - Work both legs strongly, the right knee above the ankle, the left leg straight
    - Work the right hip back and the left hip forward to square your hips
    - Lift the pelvic floor, brace the lower abdomen
    - Shoulders down, neck long, now look straight ahead
- Inhale come up, arms up if you can or lower them shoulder height
- Exhaling, change sides, adjust your feet, arms up, gaze to your thumbs
    - Breathe fully feeling your chest move, listen to your breath
    - Bend deeply into the front leg, the knee above your ankle
    - Extend out through your back leg, push out through the heel
    - Square your hips, the left hip works back, the right forward
    - Draw your shoulder down, lift your chin, soft gaze

[If necessary, do with them, face-on]
- Now, inhaling lower your arms down over your feet, open your hips and shoulders
- Exhaling open your back foot, widen the stance slightly, gaze to your left hand
    - Again we work *Virabhadrasana B* for 5 breaths
    - Your knee is above your ankle, not beyond, forward, or behind it
    - Work the knee back to open your hips and groins
    - Keep equal grounding through the right foot, especially the little toe side
    - Sit the buttocks down, sit up with your torso

	<ul><li>Inhale come up and swivel your feet to change sides</li><li>Exhaling, bend the right knee to above your ankle, gaze to the right hand<ul><li>Again sit down deeply but keep a sense of buoyancy under your hips</li><li>Both legs work strongly, the four corners of the feet grounding</li><li>Lift the pelvic floor, brace your lower belly</li><li>Breath fully into your chest, the ribs floating as you breath</li><li>Shoulders down, the front and back of the heart open</li></ul></li><li>Inhaling turn to face your right foot (come onto the back toes)</li><li>Exhale, (hands to the floor) step back to Rod</li><li>Inhale knees clear the floor, strong legs to Upward Dog</li><li>Exhale buttocks up into Downward Dog</li><li>Inhale come to your knees and relax</li></ul>

Vinyasa – Hopping to Sitting

Overview	<ul><li>**Remind of progression from Basic to Stepping in *Vinyasa***<ul><li>**Re-demonstrate both Basic and Stepping**</li></ul></li><li>**Demonstrate hopping version**</li><li>**Workshop any areas as necessary** – See script week 5</li><li>**Get them to practice**<ul><li>**Give them the option to use whichever version suits them**</li></ul></li></ul>
Introduction	<ul><li>So far we've learnt two versions of how to transit from Downward Dog to sitting in our *Vinyasa*</li><li>Just as we have gone from stepping to hopping in our sun salutation and standing postures, if you would like a further challenge in your *Vinyasa*, I'll show you the next progression – last one I promise!</li></ul>
Demonstrate side-on	<ul><li>So this is what we have done so far<ul><li>**[Demonstrate Basic *Vinyasa*]**</li></ul></li><li>Last week we kept our knees off the floor and used our arms to pull us through<ul><li>**[Demonstrate Stepping]**</li></ul></li><li>This time we do the same thing but simply hop our feet up to that position<ul><li>**[Demonstrate Stepping]**</li></ul></li></ul>
Do With / Watch Them	<ul><li>So back into Downward Dog<ul><li>At the end of your exhalation, bend your knees and look to your thumbs</li><li>Keep breathing and</li><li>Inhale, hop up, feet pointed, knees up between your hands</li><li>Keep the knees close together</li></ul></li></ul>

	o Pull your legs through
	    ▪ If you don't make it
	    ▪ Knees down, flex your feet and gently push back onto your buttocks
	        - Play with that a couple of times in your own time

REVISION: *Dandasana & Pashimottanasana A & B*		*drishti:* **toes**

Overview	• **Re-demonstrate** *Dandasana* • **Watch them do the posture** • **Workshop anything that needs refining** – See week 5 script

Demonstrate side-on	• So we go straight into our first seated posture, *Dandasana*, 'the staff'
	  o Remember *Dandasana* is like a seated *Samasthiti*
	
	Dandasana
	• Legs straight out in front
	• Arms extended down by our sides
	• We hold *Dandasana* for 5 breaths
	• From here, we go straight into our two seated forward bends
	  o Remember, all the same principles apply as when we do this posture standing
	Pashimottanasana A
	• Inhale
	• Exhale, forward, pick up the toes
	  o [Bend your knees]
	• Inhale, lift
	• Exhale into *Pashimottanasana A*
	  o 5 breaths, gazing to the toes
	• Inhale, lift up
	Pashimottanasana B
	• Exhale, hold the outside of the feet
	• Inhale, lift
	• Exhale, fold forward for 5 more breaths
	  o Let's see you do it

Do With / Watch Them	• Sit upright onto your sit bones and feel them heavy towards the floor • If you need bend the knees slightly to maintain some curve in your low back/ to keep your belly kissing your thighs • Extend out through the base of your toes and heels • Strong legs, soften your groins • Ground your hands beside your hips and lift your heart • Use a light sweeping-back action with your hands to draw your chest forward • Keep the back of the chest broad and open • Shoulder draw away from the ears as you grow tall • Lengthen your spine and neck, drop the chin

	• Gaze softly towards the tip of the nose • Breathe into all four areas of your chest listening to its sound

**Do With /
Watch Them**
	Pashimottanasana A
	• Maintaining the principles of *Dandasana*
	• Inhale lift up out of your hips
	• Exhale fold forward, pick up your big toes, bend the knees if you need
	• Inhale lift your heart, shoulders down and
	• Exhale fold forward, gazing up to your toes
	    o Extend out through the four corners of your feet
	    o Spread your sit bones wide
	    o Draw your shoulders down away from your ears
	    o Drop the chin to soften your throat
	    o Lengthen the back of your neck
	
	Pashimottanasana B
	• Inhale, lift your heart
	• Exhale, take hold of the outside edges of your feet
	• Inhale, lift broad shoulders
	• Exhale, fold forward
	    o Work your heart forward towards your feet
	    o Work up to a gentle stretch into the back of your thighs
	    o Deepen and soften the groins
	    o Lengthen through your entire spine
	    o Heart remains lifted, gaze softly to the feet

REVISION: *Purvottanasana*	*drishti:* nose or between the eyebrows

Overview	• **Re-demonstrate *Purvottanasana*** • **Briefly workshop arms, legs & neck** • **Watch them do *Purvottanasana*** • **Workshop as necessary** – See week 5 script
Introduction	• The next posture, *Purvottanasana* is the counter posture to our forward bends • I'll demonstrate it to remind you
Demonstrate side-on	• From sitting the legs are straight out in front of you • Lean back onto the hands • Inhale, lift the chest • Exhale, ground the feet • Inhale, lift the hips • Chin to the chest or head hangs back o [1 or 2 two breaths] • Exhale come down, hips first

Do With / Watch Them	<ul><li>Position your hands<ul><li>One hands length back away from our hips</li><li>The fingers point back towards you</li></ul></li><li>Straighten your arms</li><li>Inhale, lift your chest high to the ceiling</li><li>Hold it up there</li><li>Strong legs, lift your kneecaps</li><li>Point your feet, press your heels down into the mat</li><li>Inhale, lift your hips</li><li>Exhale, keep your chin on your chest or take your head back and let it hang there<ul><li>Gaze softly towards the tip of your nose</li><li>Keep the heels pressing down</li><li>Work the feet towards the floor</li><li>Strongly pull your feet towards your hands</li><li>Keep the chest high</li></ul></li><li>With an exhalation bring your hips down, the rest follows</li></ul>

Vinyasa – Hopping Back from Sitting

Overview	<ul><li>**Remind of progression from Basic to Stepping in *Vinyasa***<ul><li>**Re-demonstrate stepping back**</li></ul></li><li>**Demonstrate hopping back**</li><li>**Workshop areas as necessary** – See week 5 script</li><li>**Get them to practice**<ul><li>**Give the option to use any version in *Vinyasa***</li></ul></li></ul>**NOTE:** A *Vinyasa* is only given between every 2nd posture
Introduction	<ul><li>Remember last week we also learnt how to transit from one sitting posture to the next.</li><li>Just as we progressed our *Vinyasa* to come to sitting from stepping to hopping we can do the same when we go from sitting back into our Rod<ul><li>I'll show you what I mean</li></ul></li></ul>
Demonstrate side-on	<ul><li>This is almost the same as what we did last week, but now we simply hop both feet back at the same time instead of stepping one at a time</li><li>Let me refresh your memory on how we did it last week<ul><li>Cross your legs, feet in close to the buttocks</li><li>Bring your hands forward of your knees and</li><li>Exhaling step back into Rod (one leg at a time)</li><li>Or if you're strong</li><li>Inhale, cross the ankles and lift the feet through</li><li>Exhaling step back to Rod</li></ul></li><li>So now I'll show you the new version<ul><li>Inhale, cross the ankles</li></ul></li></ul>

	<ul><li>○ Hands forward or the knees</li><li>○ Exhale hop back (both feet together)</li><li>○ Or if you can</li><li>○ Cross and lift the feet through and</li><li>○ Exhale hop back</li></ul><ul><li>Again it is important to keep the weight forward in your hands</li><li>And to land with the low belly firm and supporting the low back</li><ul><li>○ Let's try that together</li></ul></ul>
Do With / Watch Them	<ul><li>○ Bring your hands forward of your knees</li><li>○ Or if you can</li><li>○ Draw your knees up to your chest</li><li>○ Ground your hands</li><li>○ Keep your shoulder blades down and onto your back</li><li>○ Slightly bend your elbows and create space under your armpits</li><li>○ Suck your feet up towards your armpits</li><ul><li>▪ And pull yourself through</li><li>▪ Hop back into a strong Rod</li><ul><li>- Try that again in your own time</li></ul></ul></ul>

REVISION: *Janu Shirshasana A*   drishti: *toes*

Overview	<ul><li>**Re-demonstrate *Janu Shirshasana A***</li><li>**Watch them do the posture**</li><li>**Workshop as necessary** – See week 5 script</li></ul>
Demonstrate face-on	<ul><li>I'll demonstrate the next new posture we did last class, *Janu Shirshasana A*</li><li>From *Dandasana*, our upright Rod</li><ul><li>○ Inhale bend up your right leg and take it out to the side</li><li>○ Exhale, square off</li><li>○ Inhale, hold the leg, lift up</li><li>○ Exhale, fold forward</li><ul><li>▪ Work for 5 breaths</li></ul><li>○ Inhale, lift</li><li>○ Exhale release and change legs</li></ul></ul>
Do With / Watch Them	<ul><li>Sit up tall in *Dandasana*</li><li>Bend up the right knee and close off the knee joint</li><li>Let your knee down to the side</li><li>Point your foot and work the sole up to face you</li><li>Now work your knee back to open your hips, maximum 90 degrees</li><li>Check that your left extended leg is working, press our through the heel and base of the toes with the foot upright</li><li>Inhale, square off your torso, lift your heart, hold your left leg</li></ul>

	- Exhale, shoulders down and tip forward from your hips
	  - We work in the posture for 5 breaths
	  - Gaze up to your toes, keeping the back of your neck long
	  - Breath fully into the whole of your chest, listening to your breath's sound
	  - Both legs are working, the right knee back, the left leg strong
	  - Keep your lower abdomen firm, try to recreate the curve in your low back
	- Inhale, lift the chest
	- Exhale, release the posture and straighten the right leg
	- Other side [repeat]

REVISON Workshop Possibilities	- **Protect the Knee**
	  - Don't forget to protect your knee by closing the knee joint
	  - Keep it closed as you take the knee out to the side
	  - Point your right foot and
	  - Work the soul of the foot up to face you
	    - Let me see you do that

REVISION: *Janu Shirshasana B*   *drishti:* toes

Overview	- **Re-demonstrate** *Janu Shirshasana B* - **Watch them do the posture** - Walk around to check their leg is in the right position - **Workshop any areas that need attention** – See week 5 script

Demonstrate face-on	- I'm sure that none of you have forgotten the B version!
	- Again from *Dandasana*
	- Inhaling bend the right knee, take it out to the side
	  - Foot flexed
	  - The knee comes in slightly
	  - Lift the hips up and forward
	  - The right heel sits in the crease of the buttocks
	- Square to the extended leg
	- Inhale, lift up
	- Exhale forward
	  - 5 breaths
	- Inhale, lift
	- Exhale release the posture and change sides

Do With / Watch Them	- Sit upright in *Dandasana* - Bend up your right knee and close off the knee joint - Let your knee down to the side - Place your flexed foot along the inside of your left leg - Work the right knee open to a maximum of 85 degrees - With an inhalation lift up your buttocks and move forward to sit on your right heel

	<ul><li>○ Heel in the crease of your buttocks</li><li>○ Adjust your foot position to get comfortable</li><li>○ Look down at your right leg and check that your thigh covers your calf/lower leg</li><li>○ Square off your torso to your left leg, check your left foot and leg are working</li></ul><ul><li>Inhale, hold your left leg, lift your heart</li><li>Exhale, tip forward at the hips<ul><li>○ Work here for 5 breaths</li><li>○ Gaze up to your toes, keeping the back of your neck long</li><li>○ Shoulders draw down away from the ears</li><li>○ Both feet and legs remain active, keep the right knee back, the left leg strong</li><li>○ Lift from the pelvic floor, the lower abdomen firm</li></ul></li><li>Inhale, lift the chest</li><li>Exhale, release the posture, straighten your right leg and let's do the other side</li><li>[Repeat on the left side]</li><li>*Vinyasa*</li></ul>

Marichyasana A   *drishti:* toes

Overview	<ul><li>**Introduce the *Marichyasana*s**</li><li>**Demonstrate the three progressions of *Marichyasana A***</li><li>**Do it with them &/or Watch them do it**</li><li>**Workshop as necessary**</li></ul>**NOTE:**<ul><li>Give the third stage of performing *Marichyasana* only if someone can do the second stage well</li><li>If possible, start to do the posture with them, then walk around and watch them, returning to finish the other side with them<ul><li>○ This will require you being wary of time and not holding them in the posture for too long</li></ul></li><li>There is no *Vinyasa* after *Marichyasana A* in this beginners program</li></ul>
Introduction	<ul><li>These next two postures we're about to learn are named after the sage, *Marichy*, who must have had a wicked sense of humour!</li><li>We learn the A and C versions and skip B because it's more difficult<ul><li>○ A is a forward bend with a handicap</li></ul></li></ul>
Demonstrate face-on	<ul><li>We'll work into *Marichyasana A* in three stages</li><li>**1st Stage**<ul><li>○ Sitting in *Dandasana*</li><li>○ Inhaling bend the right knee and place the foot in line with your right sit bone<ul><li>▪ To get the correct distance</li><li>▪ Spread your hand wide</li></ul></li></ul></li></ul>

	- **[Hold your hand up to demonstrate]**
	- And place your hand between your thigh and foot
	    o Inhale hug the knee up with both hands and sit up tall
	        - Try to straighten your low back / take any sag out of your low back
	    o Work your right knee back toward your armpit
	
	- **2nd Stage**
	    o If you feel you could work deeper into the posture
	    o Inhale lift up out of your hips and
	    o Exhale move your trunk forward, hands to the floor, outside your foot and leg
	    o Or you can reach one arm forward and hold your leg
	    o Notice that the buttock of your bent leg will come off the floor
	
	- **3rd Stage**
	    o Again if you feel you could go deeper
	    o Wrap your right arm around your bent leg,
	    o Wrap your left arm wraps around to meet it and clasp your hands
	    o Inhale, lift your heart
	    o Exhale, release the posture and change sides
	- We work whichever variation for 5 breaths
	- So again we have the 1st stage, 2nd and 3rd
	- **[Re-demonstrate each]**
	- Whichever stage you choose to hold and work in, try to maintain the integrity of the posture – low back not rounded, right foot grounded, heart lifted, shoulders down, etc
	    o Let's do it together

Do With / Watch Them	**1st Stage**
	- Siting in *Dandasana*
	- Bend up your right knee and place your foot at the base of your sit bone
	    o Everyone hold up your right hand
	    o Spread your fingers wide and
	    o Place your hand between your foot and your thigh
	- Inhale, hug your right leg up with both hands, lift your heart
	    o Shoulders down
	    o Ground your the right foot
	    o Continue to work out through the left foot
	    o Both legs working
	    o Work the curve back into your low back
	
	2nd Stage
	- If that feels very easy
	- Inhale lift up out of your hips and
	- Exhale, keeping the integrity of your posture, place your hands to the floor, as far back as you can
	- Or hold your leg with your right hand
	- Otherwise maintain the first posture
	    o Keep breathing fully and work your right knee back with your right arm
	    o Work your heart forward, shoulders down, heart lifted

	<ul><li>○ Tip the hips forward and splay your sit bones wide</li><li>○ The buttock of your bent leg clears the floor as you progress further forward</li></ul>**3rd Stage**<ul><li>If you feel you can work deeper forward</li><li>Inhale, reach your right arm low down around the bent knee</li><li>Exhale take your left hand behind your back, join your hands if you can<ul><li>○ Gaze up to your toes, keeping the back of your neck long</li><li>○ Remember to breath into all four areas of your chest, listening to your breath</li><li>○ Both legs are working, the right knee stays back, the left leg strong</li><li>○ Keep your lower abdomen firm, try to recreate the curve in your low back</li></ul></li><li>Inhale, lift the chest</li><li>Exhale, release the posture, straighten your right leg and we'll do the other side</li><li>[Repeat on the left side]</li></ul>
Workshop	<ul><li>**Foot Position [Demonstrate face-on]**<ul><li>○ It's important that you have your foot far enough away from your other leg so you have enough space to move forward</li><li>○ The foot is actually at hip width<ul><li>▪ Check that your hand, with your fingers spread wide, can easily fit between your thigh and foot</li></ul></li><li>○ Note that your right sit bone will come off the floor in this posture<ul><li>▪ Let's try that</li></ul></li></ul></li></ul>

Marichyasana C *drishti:* **toes**

Overview	<ul><li>**Introduce *Marichyasana C***</li><li>**Demonstrate**</li><li>**Do the posture with them/ Watch them do it**</li><li>**Workshop if necessary**</li></ul>**NOTE:**<ul><li>The hips are not square in this posture</li><li>Students do not bind *Marichyasana C* in the level 1 beginners</li><li>In the demonstration give different instructions for each side</li><li>If you do the posture with them, check that when you twist you will be able to see them (facing them)</li><li>If possible, start to do the posture with them, then hop up, walk around and watch them, then return to finish the other side with them<ul><li>○ This will require you being wary of time and not getting distracted and holding them for too long in the posture</li></ul></li><li>Both sit bones do remain grounded in *Marichyasana C*</li><li>*Vinyasa* after *Marichyasana C*</li></ul>

Introduction	• *Marichyasana C* is a seated twist ○ Watch me do it first

Demonstrate
 	
Bent knee side-on
	• From *Dandasana*
	• Inhaling bend up your right knee
	• Exhaling twist to face the bent knee
	• Right hand close to your buttocks
	• Left elbow to the outside of your right knee
	   ○ 5 breaths here, gazing right
	• Inhale, undo the twist
	• Exhale, release the posture, change sides
	• Note that in *Marichyasana C* the foot is in close to the thigh
	• Lift out of your hips to twist
	• Right hand supports you, opposite elbow to knee
	• 5 breaths
	• Inhale look back to the foot
	• Exhale and release
	   ○ Let's do that together / Let me see you do it

**Do With /
Watch Them**
	• Sitting upright in *Dandasana*
	• With an inhalation bend up your right knee, your foot in close to your thigh
	• Lift up out of your hips and twist at your waist
	• Exhale, place the right hand close to the base of your spine
	• The outside of your left elbow to the outside of your knee
	   ○ Hold *Marichyasana C* for 5 breaths, gazing to the right
	   ○ Lightly press your elbow against your knee and
	   ○ At the same time work your knee back against your elbow
	      ▪ This will maintain the position of the knee above the ankle
	   ○ Ground both sit bones toward the floor and lengthen your spine
	   ○ Work the shoulders open/away from each other
	   ○ Keep the back of the neck lengthening
	   ○ Gaze softly over your right shoulder
	• Inhale, look back to your left foot, check that it is upright
	• Exhale, release the posture and change sides
	• Inhale, left foot in close to the left thigh, the hips unlevel
	• Exhale, twist, place the left hand behind you, right elbow to left knee
	• Inhale, lift out of your hips and twist the shoulders further left
	   ○ Take 5 full breaths, maintaining the knee above the ankle
	   ○ Sit down through the sit bones, sit up out of your hips
	   ○ Lift your heart, shoulders down, long spine, long neck
	   ○ Chase the left shoulder back as you gaze toward it
	   ○ Continue to work the left, straight leg
	   ○ Lightly press the elbow against the knee to work deeper in the posture
	• Inhale look back to your right foot
	• Exhale and release the posture
	• ***Vinyasa***

| Workshop | **Unlevel hips**
• As we twist, the hips will want to unlevel/become unsquared
• Allow this to happen as most of the rotation should happen in the chest portion of the spine
    o The vertebrae in your low back are not designed to twist

Foot position
• The foot is in closer than *Marichyasana A*
    o The closer the foot to the thigh, the easier it is to twist
    o With the foot out wider you will need to twist further

Knee position
• You can take your knee across your midline to enter the posture, and then reposition the knee above the ankle
• Work to maintain the position of your knee above the ankle
    o To do this you need to have an arm wrestle between your elbow and your knee - with neither one winning!
        ▪ Lightly press your elbow against your knee and
        ▪ At the same time work your knee back against your elbow
• This action will also help you to work deeper into the twist

Lift your heart
• Maintain the integrity of your upper body posture
• Do not sacrifice this to get deeper into the twist or you will lose the benefits of the posture
    o Ground your sit bones and, at the same time, lift up out of your hips
    o Keep the heart lifted, shoulders down, the entire spine and neck lengthening |

Navasana	*drishti:* **toes**
Overview	• **Introduce *Navasana*** • **Demonstrate with bent knees** o **Show full version** • **Do it with them once** • **Watch them do it twice** • **Workshop if necessary** **NOTE:** • Keep breaths/ instructions short as this is a strenuous posture • Give beginners one breaths break between each repetition • Beginners only do three repetitions of *Navansana*
Introduction	• Our last new posture is *Navasana*, or the boat posture o Our word 'navy' comes from the *Sanskrit Nava,* which means boat • In this posture we should resemble a boat

Demonstrate side-on	**Knees Bent**
	• From *Dandasana*, lean back
	• Inhale, pick up your feet
	• Arms extended
	   o 5 breaths here
	• Exhale, feet down and
	• Inhaling buttocks up
	• Exhale down
	   o We repeat this three times
	
	Full Version
	• If you can keep your back straight and your heart lifted
	   o You can straighten out your legs
	      ▪ Let's do one together

Do With / Watch Them	• Siting upright in *Dandasana*
	• Bend your knees
	• Now lean back to a comfortable position
	   o Behind your sit bones and in front of your tailbone
	• Inhaling, pick up your feet
	• Extend your arms out straight, knee height and parallel to the floor
	• Palms facing each other
	• We work for 5 breaths here
	   o Gaze softly to your toes
	   o Continue to lift your heart
	   o Shoulders down
	   o Work towards having your shins parallel to the floor
	   o Don't clench your jaw – it won't help
	• Exhale, lower your feet, cross your ankles
	• Inhale, lift your hips up into your armpits
	• Exhale, lower down
	• Inhale hug your knees up to your chest and release your low back
	   o I'll watch you do the next two
	   o Brace your lower abdomen
	   o Work as if to keep the curve in your low back
	   o Knees together
	   o Feet together and pointed
	   o Relax your jaw and face
	   o Long neck
	   o Drop your chin
	   o Lengthen through the crown of your head

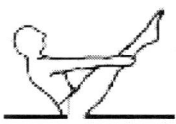

Shavasana	
Overview	**NOTE:** • The following *Shavasana* is more suited to the final class(es) of a beginners course or more advanced classes • Offer students an eye pillow • Once you have students relaxed do not move, shuffle papers or

	- make any noise – be still and quiet yourself
- Adjust your tone and pace to induce a state of relaxation
- Be sure to vary your words: relax, soften, release, let go, etc
- At the end, taper off your instruction, making it clear that you are finished
- Get students out of relaxation with a quiet, slow voice or gently use chimes or chant
- At the end remember to remind students to neatly fold and stack their blankets
	- Prepare yourself for *Shavasana*
- Make yourself totally comfortable
- Everyone, take a big breath in and let it all out
- Completely let go of any control of your breath, let it fall to normal, whatever that is for you right now
- Let your whole body fall heavy onto the mat
- Soften all of your joints
- And feel all your muscle relax and let go
- Check that your feet are relaxed and that your ankles and knees are loose and soft
- Relax all of the muscles in the front and back of your legs
- Feel your buttocks and the back of your legs where they touch the floor and let them fall heavy onto the mat
- Release and soften your hips and lower abdomen
- Feel the length of your spine relax, including your neck
- The shoulders fall open, the arms and hands melt as if they were liquid
- The chest relaxed, the ribs soft and loose
- Let your face soften, your brow smooth
- With the whole of your body totally relaxed, now also let go of your awareness of your body
- Leave it lying there relaxed on the mat
- Instead, draw your attention inward
- Behind your closed eyes, look at the vast space existing inside you
- Give yourself the space to develop your insight and perception
- Deafen your ears to the sounds outside of you and instead listen to the quiet and the stillness that exists inside
- Take the time to listen to your inner voice, your true self
- And feel your breath as it comes and goes
- Notice how effortlessly the breath enters you, without any conscious effort on your part
- And how it automatically exits, leaving you with the gift of life
- Feel yourself being breathed
- Being sustained with every breath
- And allow yourself to trust, to completely let go, 100 per cent
- **Chant** or **Chimes**
- Gently bring your awareness back into the room
- Back into your body
- Begin to move your fingers and toes
- When you're ready, bend up your knees and roll over onto one side
- Rest there for a moment then slowly and in your own time come up to sitting